C

Medical Blunders

Medical Blunders

Robert M. Youngson
&
Ian Schott

NEW YORK UNIVERSITY PRESS
Washington Square, New York

First published in the U.S.A. in 1996 by
NEW YORK UNIVERSITY PRESS
Washington Square
New York, N.Y. 10003

Library of Congress Cataloging-in-Publication Data

Youngson, R. M.
    Medical blunders : amazing true stories of mad, bad, and dangerous doctors /
Robert M. Youngson and Ian Schott.
        p.   cm.
    Includes index.
    ISBN 0-8147-9678-8
    1. Medical errors. 2. Quacks and quackery. I. Schott, Ian. II. Title.
R729.8.Y68   1996   96—15294
610—dc20   CIP

Printed in Great Britain

Contents

Preface

'Trust me, I'm a doctor' has been the message of the medical fraternity down the ages. And impressed by their apparent ability to understand the hidden mysteries of the body, and the even more hidden matters of the mind, the vast majority of people have indeed trusted them. Patients have been amazingly patient, acting as human 'guinea pigs', submitting themselves to the knife, to noxious medicines, to ordeals of both a physical and a psychological nature.

But how much do doctors really know? And how often is the patient's trust abused by quacks or incompetents? Robert M. Youngson and Ian Schott have produced a gripping selection of the worst frauds, blunders and abuses perpetrated over the centuries in the name of medicine - a horribly fascinating account of wrong thinking and wrongdoing from the Ancient Greeks to the wilder shores of the contemporary medical scene.

Robert M. Youngson, a doctor himself, says that although doctors are in general more careful than other people, cases of mishap and malpractice, from wrong dosages to the removal of perfectly healthy parts of the body, do occur in everyday medicine, while professional arrogance and ambition have led to transgressions from some of the most eminent names in the medical research field. Ian Schott is an experienced investigative journalist, who makes it his business to uncover fraud and expose incompetence. Occasionally names and details have had to be altered to protect patients still living who would not wish to be identified, but all the stories included in the book are true, in that the events actually happened, and many have been previously reported in the medical press.

Chapter One

Famous quacks & infamous cures

Film-O-Sonics, and other miracles of technology

The Golden Age of what might be called 'pseudo-technological quackery' was the period following the end of the Second World War. Throughout the Deep South and the west coast of America, there appeared a species of ingenious medical entrepreneur. From the early 1950s a range of exotic-looking devices, covered with a profusion of knobs, flashing lights and spurious dials, came on the market. Pride of place among all these imaginative products of human chicanery should go to the 'Film-O-Sonic', the invention of a San Bernadino chiropractor and a bargain at $500. To a casual observer, this might have looked like a primitive tape recorder with the speaker removed (which in fact it was). While a mysterious tape played in the machine (which no one could hear, there being no speaker), pads attached to the device were applied to the body to expel cancer, cataracts, heart diseases and ulcers. So what was on this tape that was so therapeutic to the patient and that made diseases so keen to flee the body? It was a loop-tape of Frank Sinatra singing 'Smoke gets in your eyes'.

Cancer-detector

Another device was that made by Mark Callert, a self-styled radon expert, lecturer and 'naturopath', in 1952. His device – a panel covered by a rash of switches and lights, all connected in electrical series – resembled the flight deck of an intergalactic cruiser. It was asserted that it could diagnose and treat tumours, cancer, syphilis and most other diseases to boot. The deluxe model sold at $545, and Callert did a brisk trade. He himself practiced with it, and added zodiacally-inspired diagnostic techniques into his patter. To reach an opinion on a patient, he stroked a metal plate on the machine; when it squeaked back at him, he pronounced judgement. To prescribe a treatment, the patient invariably being told that he was gravely ill, Callert placed a number of bottles of coloured water on the machine, and invited it to select one, which it did by means of a flashing bulb. Within a short time, Callert established a thriving practice, until he unfortunately told an unusually healthy federal investigator that he was afflicted by 'cancer of the liver, a tumour pressing on the heart and lymphogranuloma.' Despite the ostentatious electrical wizardry of the machine, it transpired that the only circuit in it was the one connecting it to the mains.

The imaginative merging of scientific technology has always been a facet of quackery. Dwellers in the twilight zone of post-war America saw the germination of a space program, the first vast, unwieldy, but impressive computers, television and tape recorders. The world moved into the nuclear age, without understanding fully the consequences of atomic radiation. It became perceived as a mystic source of power, whose destructiveness bore witness to the miraculous good it might produce if harnessed differently. The curious militant aspect of technology was reflected in the weird and wonderful death-rays and space-rockets that filled the paranoid fiction of the time, in which small-town America was constantly threatened by blobs of alien goo, body-snatching plants and creatures that burrowed in under one's skin and consumed the human brain. Like disease, these creatures threatened the health of every American. In the films they were fought with ingenious technology. People began to look for suitable space-age weapons to fight their own sicknesses, cancer in particular.

Callert's device was highly influential in this sphere, and spawned such imitators as 'Ralph R. Rueber's Analyzer', which was rather more compact, consisting of three electrical circuits which lit up two bulbs and warmed a plate which was stroked to reach a diagnosis. Rueber also produced an 'Energiser', which was very similar except for the peculiar addition of a couple of pounds of tar.

The McCoy Device

Other unusual diagnostic machines included the 'McCoy Device', which was popular in San José in 1951. McCoy, an oil dealer, created a machine which deduced the nature of ailments from the patient's signature. Clients then had to undergo at least ninety days' treatment on his 'Oscilloclast' at, at least, $1 a day, after which the state of their signature would indicate that they were cured. Six years of technological advancement later, 'Dr' Newfield produced 'Dr John Sumner Newfield's Electro-Metabiograph Diagnostic Machine and Quantimeter', which retailed at $250 and could diagnose and cure heart diseases, high blood pressure and prostate gland disorders.

Radiation fascinated people. They had a vague notion that it might produce terrible mutations, but they believed that used correctly it was a wonder cure for cancer. People paid $200 a day to sit in old radium mines, and paid hundreds more dollars to attend one of a series of 'Uranium Centers' set up in 1953 in northern California. In these, they lay in cubicles lined with low-grade uranium ore, or on beds with trays of uranium under them, hopefully exposing themselves to hideous doses of radiation in the belief that it would destroy cancer and arthritis.

The Radon Generator

If you couldn't make it to one of these fashionable resorts, you could manufacture your own radioactive water at home, and were recommended to drink several gallons of it a day. A range of useful kitchenware was available, advertised in newspapers and peddled door to door. The 'Radon Generator', a bullet-shaped capsule about three inches tall, which its inventors claimed contained $4,000 worth of high-grade radium chloride, was designed to be put in a thermos jug of tap water, which would then be drunk to cure each and every human sickness. In addition, it revived wilted flowers. Fortunately for the purchasers, it was found to contain $1.30 worth of radium. Alternatively, you could buy the 'Radon Magic Cure-All Jug'. This essential item was a two-gallon pitcher with a silver-coloured bell attached to a stick on the lid. Lowered into the jug, the bell transformed ordinary tap water into a tasty, hot 'n' spicy radioactive brew which it was said would have a miraculous effect on cancer, rheumatic fever, baldness and general vitality.

For those undecided as to whether they should spend their money on their health or a useful piece of furniture, why not invest $300 in the 'Atomitron'? In 1954, over thirty of the good folk of Texas did. At first glance this was an ordinary and really rather shoddy kitchen sideboard, available only in white formica. When you opened the doors, however, you could see where the money went. It was fitted with a sun lamp, two milk bottles, a short-wave receiver and a variety of coloured slides. This device would, if the instructions were followed, attract 'short-wave radiation' and fill one bottle with 'E' water, bubbling with beneficial electrons, and the other with 'T' water, for 'thermal energy'. It was sold as a 'major contribution to the welfare of mankind' and its produce was recommended for all major afflictions, including cancer, tumours, apoplexy and ulcers. 'It combines,' read the sales pitch, 'the four sciences of chromology [*sic*], electronics, hydroponics and ethereal atoms.' For some unknown reason the customisation of the sideboard was completed by turning the top drawer upside down.

'Rays'

'Rays' – sound, radio and light – held something of the mystery of radiation, and it was popularly believed that they could be beamed at invasive diseases with devastating results; all one needed was the correct weapon with which to harness their power. From this assumption arose the 'Gravitronic Life-Ray Table', the 'only cure for cancer,' which shot radio waves, altered by a secret process, at the patient, and 'stimulated the cancer germs to death.' The machine was a tape recorder with a nasty shock hazard due to faulty wiring.

There was also a fashion for having an ozone generator in the living room – not an advisable purchase – and several thousand versions of the 'Calozone', 'Orozone', 'Neurozone' and 'Airozone' machines were sold throughout the West Coast at up to $200 a time. The Californian market was particularly fruitful for this techno-quackery because of its affluence, the traditional interest of its inhabitants in their health, and the age of the population; retired, wealthy people, with the resources to indulge their multifarious health concerns, moved to California in droves after the Second World War, and those over sixty-five made up 10 per cent of the population by the early 1960s.

Quacks & the niche market

Quacks have always had an eye for the niche market. The old are a traditional prey, but additionally there have always been conditions which it has not been considered suitable to address publicly, syphilis or impotence, for example; latterly, cancer and AIDS have a similar stigma attached to them. Quacks identify these areas of fear and ignorance, and mine them ruthlessly with very specific marketing techniques. These are the highly lucrative areas of quackery. Now the modern pharmaceutical industry is equally selective about the drugs it develops, targeting those diseases which are likely to prove most financially rewarding. Third World diseases are of less interest to drug companies than the ulcers caused by the Western lifestyle, for example. Ulcers are a chronic condition; they stay, the patient becomes a regular customer, the company's long-term income is assured. Third World populations can't necessarily pay the bills.

Another historic characteristic of quackery is its self-advertisement. Indeed, 'quack' is an abbreviation of a Dutch word, 'quacksalver', meaning, literally, 'he who quacks about his salves.' This reliance on advertising has traditionally outraged established medical practitioners and has been used as a rule to discriminate between the genuine doctor and the quack. The genuine medical practitioner has no need to sell himself; he is quietly confident of his resources, and furthermore, to advertise would be to bid for ill-health. Truth is modest. By contrast, the quack has no qualms; he competes shamelessly, he advertises, he sells door to door and from a showman's stage, making claims which the orthodox doctor cannot respectably match.

In the seventeenth and eighteenth centuries, when medicine was still largely theoretical and qualifications often a matter of simple agreement with current ideas, there was little difference between the effectiveness of the quack and the established doctor; the patient stood an equal chance of being poisoned by either. Quackery became a term for unwanted competition; the quack was always someone else. Quackery was, in a manner, the creation of scholastic medicine, with its clinical schools and qualifications and institutions deciding what was acceptable, and what was forbidden; the quack was the mountebank, the showman, the outsider, the aggressive buccaneer of the free market. Doctors, a most conservative bunch with their silver-topped canes and frock coats, had invested heavily in their costly 'education' and were financially dependent on annexing exclusive access to the wealthy; they invoked the horror of the quack and in particular the vulgarity of quack advertising in defence of their desire for a closed shop. Johnson's *Dictionary* of 1755 virtually defines the quack in terms of his use of publicity; the quack is a 'vain, boastful pretender to physic, one who proclaims his own medical abilities in public places.'

Orthodox and unorthodox schools
In reality there was little difference between the orthodox and

unorthodox schools of medicine. They shared the same basic language, and the belief that the body was composed of a mixture of solids, fluids and 'humours' and that disease occurred as a consequence of the imbalance of these. In many ways quacks, often adept at tooth-pulling and the setting of broken bones, were of more practical use than their established compatriots. Their methods could be based more on experience than theory, and could consequently be more directly effective. The accepted and thoroughly toxic medicines of the orthodox pharmacopoeia were used by both sides. Opiates, mercury mixtures and doses of antimony (a potentially lethal metallic compound) were given liberally. Nor were the quacks illegal; it would have been hard to identify whom one was legislating against, since quackery seemed to be judged either subjectively, or on the basis of the amount and style of publicity employed by a practitioner. Indeed, 'quack' was a term that could be applied to anyone showing suspect ambition in their professional field. 'We have,' wrote Tobias Smollett, 'quacks in religion, quacks in physic, quackery in law, quacks in politics, quacks in patriotism, quacks in government.'

It was not until the Apothecaries Act of 1815 and the Medical Registration Act of 1858 that any clear regulations regarding entitlement to practice emerged.

Georgian England provided an excellent market place for the aggressive health practitioner (it seems more representative to term him that than 'quack'). While the growth of the mercantile middle classes meant that there was a lot more wealth around to pursue, there were still plague and smallpox to be 'cured', and ignorance of hygiene (pus was still thought 'noble', and sanitation was still elementary) ensured the continuation of real sickness in the population. As people became greater consumers of goods generally, they also began to buy more products which they thought beneficial to health. They were testing the power of their new wealth. People bought ready-made consumer items that they had previously manufactured at home or gone without: candles, beer, soap, ironmongery. But the new wonder was the pill. It was bought by the hundreds of thousands, or simply by weight, and gulped by the handful.

This was the age of the spa, when the middle classes would retire to Bath, or Buxton, or Tunbridge Wells to take the waters; it became an age of fashionable hypochondria, of listlessness, of 'the vapours', of physical overindulgence and faintness, nervous disorder and biliousness; of a whole range of imaginary social diseases to be treated in entertaining ways, in addition to the upsurge of the venereal diseases, syphilis and gonorrhoea.

Pride of place among the respectable family's possessions were the medicine chests – one for the gentlemen, one for the ladies and a third for the horses – stuffed with over a hundred of the latest pills, potions and doses from reputable practitioner and quack alike. Everybody swigged and swallowed; self-treatment was a hobby; tomes on treating oneself poured off the press:*Every Man His Own Physician*, *The Complete Family Physician*. People kept diaries of their experiments with drugs, and swapped notes on experiences. 'When I took Mrs Stephen's Medicines,' wrote the Reverend Edmund Pyle with great composure, 'I swallowed two ounces of soap a day, for six months together. Besides the oystershell, or eggshell powder, in small beer. I think the doses were three or four in a day.'

No doubt Mrs Stephen's Medicines were highly expensive

as well. The average 'nostrum' – a dose of one of these medicines – might cost a shilling, a day's wage for a labourer, or two or three shillings for a bottle. 'Kennedy's Lisbon Diet Drink', a discreet and ineffective cure for syphilis, cost half a guinea for a bottle, and you were required to drink two bottles a day. The English became fascinated with sickness, addicted to self-drugging.

The rise of brand name medicines

It was the healthy state of the printed word that gave birth to advertising and provided the means to reach and develop the tastes of the public. It came principally in the shape of hand-bills and in advertisements placed in the new medium of news-papers, which provided an excellent stimulus to sales. Handbills were not only thrust at people on the streets but were left in libraries and bookshops. Rising literacy levels helped to create the market for commercial medicine, bookshops even providing sales outlets for pills. The learned style or sheer lin-guistic verve of the handbills seduced the public. One typical handbill of 1677, headed 'The Woman's Prophecy or the Rare and Wonderful Doctrines,' offered to cure 'The Glimmering of the Gizard, the Quavering of the Kidneys and the Wambling Trot.' Others overwhelmed the reader with intricate stories about the origin of a complaint, linking the specific illness to a general, vague dysfunctioning of the body for which the adver-tised product was the sole cure: 'The scurvy is a certain evil habit of the whole body turning all the ailment we receive into evil humours taking its original from Crude and Melancholy Humours, the Cause whereof is for want of good Digestion in the stomach caused either by obstructions of the Spleen, or Liver and Sometime from the Obstruction of the Sweetbreads and also from a raw and undigested Blood in the whole Body, but chiefly in the Hypochondries or Sides, which offends by a certain specific Putrefaction arising from our Diet ...'

Brand names emerged, established in the public memory through handbills and labels: 'Doctor James's Powders', 'Anderson's Scots Pill', 'Hooper's Female Pills', 'Doctor Radcliffe's Famous Purging Elixir', 'Turlington's Pills', 'Bateman's Pectoral Drops', 'Daffy's Elixir'. Sales rocketed, and in spite of public protestations that the public were being thoroughly gulled by quacks, many established medical figures were also making a killing with named brands and nostrums.

Joshua Ward
Unqualified medical practitioners with charm and verve rose rapidly through the ranks of society. Joshua Ward, who made a vast profit from the sale of his Pill and Drop, was knighted after he successfully twiddled with George II's dislocated thumb. His products became standard issue for the British Navy and he amassed enough wealth to endow four London hospitals for the poor, at which his products were to be liberally used, thus ensuring his prosperity.

William Read, whom Joseph Addison called 'the most laborious advertiser of his time,' began life as a tailor but became a self-taught oculist and after treating Queen Anne received the customary knighthood and dwelt thereafter among the glamorous literati of the day.

'Piss Prophets' were those who dealt in uroscopy, the process of divining sickness from urine. Although there continues to be a valid medical foundation to this process, urine has few of the extraordinary powers then attributed to it.

Urine was particularly useful in the diagnosis of real or

imagined syphilis. God help the unfortunate who gave an acquisitive doctor a urine sample: he would discover that he had every conceivable sexual complaint, and it would cost him dear if he wanted to live.

The same was still true thirty years into Queen Victoria's reign. Sexual problems did not receive a wide public airing in the Victorian world, despite the proliferation of prostitution, syphilis and gonorrhoea. Syphilis, with its terrifying tertiary stage of madness and physical putrefaction, was dreaded. For a long time the only commonly-known treatment for it was mercury, which caused fever and excessive salivation, swollen glands, loose teeth and a fetid body odour. In short, it was impossible to conceal from one's nearest and dearest that one was undergoing treatment for syphilis; men would gladly undergo any sort of alternative treatment in an effort to conceal the result of their infidelities from their wives. While the brains of the most famous and brilliant rotted away, robust ideas of Christian manly vigour were publicly promulgated. Impotence, wet dreams and masturbation were all believed to be fatal symptoms of hopeless moral and physical decay, of femininity, possibly of some terrible disease. The Victorians regarded the undirected loss of sperm with horror.

The Medical Registration Act of 1858
So the unqualified, aggressive medical practitioners, who by 1858 had been prevented from competing in the open market-place by the Medical Registration Act, which allowed only quacks certified by the establishment to practice, began to focus on these areas in which public ignorance prevailed. Their activities thrived. In 1865, there was a veritable ring of them practicing in London. Some used a number of names and

addresses to maintain several practices simultaneously. They left handbills and posters in public toilets and advertised their services in newspapers by inviting the reader to send away for books with oblique titles such as *Manly Vigour* or *The Philosophy of Marriage*, books which would emphasize the danger to one's strength and sanity posed by nocturnal emissions. There was a phenomenal amount of such advertising, and the quacks would shamelessly quote from their previous advertisements in other newspapers in such a way that it appeared that their publications had been favourably reviewed by those newspapers. Here is an excerpt from *Manhood: A Medical Essay* by Dr Curtis (alias J. La Mert) of 15 Albermarle St, Piccadilly: 'On the cause and cure of Premature Decline in Man. The Treatment of the nervous and physical debility, loss of memory and muscular power, pains in the back and those diseases which tend to embitter and shorten life.'

While purporting to give reassuring advice to those wondering what precisely was supposed to be happening between the sheets, these books confronted young men with the abject shame of their inadequacies. As Dr Walter de Roos of Bloomsbury Square wrote in his informative *The Medical Advisor:* 'What mockery more deep than the desolation of spirit which an affectionate woman must feel on finding that she clasps within her circling embrace the mere wreck of sensualism of the debilitated victim of self-pollution, one who having unduly or precociously exercised his imagination and bodily powers is now deprived of that capability for which his genitive organs were destined.'

The message was clear: masturbation ruined your life, and even involuntary dribbling in your sleep was likely to cause madness. The concerned reader was generally invited to visit the doctor, if distance made this inconvenient, to send a urine sample by post. The urine sample invariably yielded the feared result: that the unfortunate reader showed evidence of 'spermattorrhea'. This could be cured. First, one must send money to buy a special support, such as Doctor Hammond's 'Self-Adjusting Curative', described as a 'small elegant, unique apparatus, adapted with exquisite accuracy to encircle the genitive organs to which is added a SAFETY VALVE which prevents and stops EMISSIONS.'

It was unlikely, the patient was generally advised by Doctor Hammond, that this customised support alone would prove sufficient. Here is a letter to an anxious provincial gentleman who corresponded with him (Hammond having no need actually to see his patients):

'I have again gone into your case and am decidedly of the opinion that the principal seat of disease is in the seminal vessels which have become greatly relaxed in their tone and power of retention. There appears also to be some slight disease of the kidneys. I am also of the opinion that the semen passes constantly away in the urine and that the result of this drain on the constitution must be obvious, when I tell you that ONE DROP OF SEMEN IS EQUAL TO FORTY DROPS OF BLOOD... should this drain of the most vital of all your secretions be not IMMEDIATELY ARRESTED, your whole system must suffer serious derangement, whilst the organs of generation themselves will relapse into a state of utter impotency. This must necessarily destroy all desire for sexual intercourse with entire loss of erectile power, WITHERING and WASTING of the penis; and in addition, afflictions of the head and INSANITY are among the first results of such a state and although you do not yet complain of such, YET HAVE YOU

REASON TO FEAR THEIR APPEARANCE ...'

The 'only' treatment for all serious cases – and all cases were serious – finally made an explicit connection in the mind of the client between his own condition and syphilis. He had already been told that his leaking sperm could send him mad; now he was informed that the only certain cure involved mercury. Mercury! The horror and shame! Into the imaginative vacuum of the client regarding his sexuality, the quack coaxed the latent terror of venereal infection; the patient realized, to his despair, that what he had was not a problem, but a disease, equivalent in its malignancy to syphilis.

Summoned to see the quack in person, to receive free advice, he would be shown a model illustrating in detail the horrible effects of the mercury treatment on the human face. There was, he would be told, an alternative, the 'gold' treatment, but it was very expensive. 'How much?' the anguished patient gasps, staring at the awful model, its distended gums, the blank holes where teeth once were, the cracked, oozing skin and collapsing syphilitic nose. 'He was a young man once,' says the quack, 'not dissimilar to yourself, and handsome too.' The young man is close to tears, 'How much?' The quack sighs and clucks as he appears to compute. 'It will cost five hundred pounds in your advanced stage of morbidity.' Five hundred pounds is a vast, impossible sum of money to the young man. He cannot afford the treatment. He weeps.

The quack appears to have an idea. He consoles his visitor. He will accept a down payment now, and then the rest will be payable in instalments, at a fixed interest rate. The young man is too relieved to notice that this is close to 400 per cent; nor, dreading publicity, will he complain. Believing himself a patient, he has become a victim of blackmail.

This did actually happen to a number of young men around this period. Fortunately, some later consulted other doctors who told them there was nothing wrong with them, and they sued successfully for the return of the vast sums they had paid for the 'gold' treatment.

Modern alternative medicine

Recent surveys in America and Britain reveal that an increasing section of the population regularly uses 'alternative' medicine. In Britain, a 1986 report found that there were 116 various alternative treatments that were consistently used, and an American study of 660 cancer patients found that over half were using alternative healing methods; some had never undertaken orthodox treatment and a substantial proportion had abandoned it in favour of alternative therapy. Is this clientele driven to the unorthodoxies of chiropracty, herbalism, acupuncture and aromatherapy by poverty or superstitious ignorance? It is an area popular with the affluent and educated middle class; it is more likely that consumers are simply disappointed with the narrow relationship they have with their doctors and with the reductive, material limits of conventional medicine. Moreover, conventional medicine puts ultimate restraints on the power of money. But in the alternative field, the wealthy can explore. An exotic profusion of Aquarian therapies arouses concern that we live in a new age of quackery, with all the fantastic elements of that tradition.

The miraculous power to heal simply through the laying on of hands has been attributed to many individuals throughout history. Often the power is an essential part of the individual's claim to divine authority, and hence the ability to heal has often been part of the public image of royalty. The British monarch traditionally claimed the right to cure scrofula (tuberculosis of the lymphatic glands) by simple application of the royal touch. This disease was known as the'King's Evil', and the monarchy was still touching people for it in the eighteenth century. It was practiced by the Saxon kings and revived by the Tudors; this was a time of great conflict over the throne, and an ability to cure scrofula was evidence of the legitimacy of one's claim. Small gold, and later silver, 'touch pieces' were also given to the public who were fanatically keen on the very grand ceremony of touching, though whether people were cured by the money or the royal digit is unclear. After the restoration of the monarchy, Charles II naturally developed the ceremony into a highly impressive demonstration of the divine powers by which he ruled; it was show business and the public adored it. William III, however, had no time for it. When he was told a vast crowd were besieging the palace at Lent, screaming to be touched, he told his staff to 'Give the poor creatures some money and send them away.' Once cornered by a grovelling supplicant begging to be touched, he reluctantly consented, saying 'God give you better health and a little intelligence.' Queen Anne was the last person to touch officially, though some of the aura surrounding the act survives in the attention given to living royals when they so much as shake the hand of a fatally sick patient.

Actually, what we have today is more complicated than simple quackery. Today's alternative therapies are something of a throwback, a mixture of mysticism, 'traditional' and natural remedies with a sprinkling of the occult. Quackery has always been at the forefront of technology. Magnetism, electricity, radiation, the first commercially produced pills – quackery has always assured people that they are getting the latest, the most sophisticated treatment. Quackery is more a collection of characteristics than individual types of treatment. These characteristics – exploitation of technology as a novelty, a reliance on advertising and the selective targeting of sickness for commercial gain – seem now, ironically, the province of mainstream commercial medicine.

Much of today's alternative medicine is claimed to be based on tradition, mystic folk remedies; but it manifests itself in homoeopathy, crystal-stroking, faith-healing and so on, treatments resorted to in sickness, whereas much of folk medicine is concerned with preventing future illness by observing rites, rituals and taboos; it is the consequence of a system of beliefs.

There are no germs, microbes, viruses or defective genes in the world of preventative folk medicine. Sickness arises as a consequence of supernatural forces. Therefore, the effects of these must be avoided by strict observance of rituals; if they cannot be averted, they must be fought by other supernatural methods. The principal three causes of disease are the anger of an offended external spirit; the supernatural powers of a human enemy; and, most importantly, the displeasure of the dead.

The first has much to do with animism, the belief that the natural world is alive with unseen intelligent spirits. It also has much to do, in Christian societies, with the Devil, who seems to be regarded as the head of the medical profession. Sir George McKenzie wrote in the seventeenth century that 'the Devil may inflict diseases which is an effect he may occasion by applying actives to passives and by the same means he may likewise cure and not only may he cure diseases laid on by himself but even natural diseases since he knows the natural causes and origins of even those natural diseases better than physicians can, who are not present when diseases are contracted and who, being younger than he must have less experience.'

Evidently a doctor's doctor, McKenzie's wilful and wise Devil would today be writing a weekly column for a Sunday newspaper. Diseases and plagues are still personified as malign, destroying angels; Death stalks the land as a skeleton; the plague is one of the horsemen of the apocalypse, or is spread by vampires.

In ancient culture there were literally thousands of spirits to pacify – the Assyrians had 900 toxic spirits that could be swallowed in food and drink alone, which bears tolerable comparison with our dread of 'E' numbers. Apart from being food additives, spirits dwelt in rivers, mountains, trees and lakes, and preventative medicine compelled one to avoid giving offence. In addition, the beneficial gods and spirits of a conquered race would become the devils plaguing their conquerors. The sorcerer, witch, charmer or wise woman brings sickness upon another human by practicing magic which may be a direct effect upon their victim; or it may actually be the spirits or the Devil who finally inflicts the disease.

For those who want to try this at home, the basic principles of traditional magic are 'sympathetic': that is, magic depends upon the mysterious sympathy between apparently disparate objects and actions. There are two branches to this: homoeopathic or imitative magic, and contagious magic. Homoeopathic magic holds that like equals like, so in order to inflict acute arthritic pain on an enemy you stick a needle into the hip of a model representing that enemy. Modern homoeopathic medicine treats diseases by administering small quantities of drugs that excite symptoms similar to those of the disease as the principle also holds that like counters like.

When extended into the realms of modern drugs this can be disastrous; for example, overdoses of barbiturate 'downers' were briefly treated with a similar overdose of barbiturate 'uppers', on the principle that one would counter the other – instead of which the patient habitually received a double overdose and died. Contagious magic holds that whatever has once been in contact with a person remains forever in contact. To practice this you will need to obtain toenails, hair clippings, used underwear or similar objects belonging to the intended victim. You then subject these to the worst possible torment you can devise. Smash their favourite records, for example. It may not have any immediate effect on them but it will make you feel much better.

Sir George McKenzie also had a highly sophisticated explanation as to how the Devil fitted into the realm of magic and disease: 'Witches do likewise torment mankind by making images of clay and wax and when the witches prick or pince these images the person whom these images represent do find extreme torment which doth not proceed from any influence these images have upon the body tormented, but the Devil doth by natural means raise these torments in the person tormented at the same time that the witches do prick or pince.'

So the magic is simply a series of coded requests to the Devil, who converts these abstract signals into real aches, pain, vomiting and fevers; the symptoms are, in themselves, natural. But disease, which otherwise must be viewed as coming without reason, explanation or justice, has an origin in sheer human malice: those damn witches, slaving away in their gloomy image factory, moulding, pricking and pinching until their hands are sore and bleeding.

The dead must not be crossed. This applied quite literally in

New England in the last century, where stepping on a grave was liable to give you a fever. Generally, the dead were potentially contagious or could inflict sickness if the correct customs and rituals were not observed towards them.

This aspect of preventative folk medicine had the potential to create social chaos in certain parts of antique Scotland and Ireland. Here it was believed that the spirit of the man most recently buried in a graveyard was condemned to watch over it until relieved from his irksome, tedious duties by the spectre of the next fatality. A dead man's relatives would be greatly concerned to think of their deceased kinsman's ghost standing out all night in the cold and rain, and would be keen to see the next corpse buried as soon as possible. Hence, in these parts of the world, one was not encouraged to save the life of a dying man because in so doing you were condemning the ghost of the last man to die to a continued wretched watch, for which he was unlikely to thank you; your good deed would be punished by vicious fevers.

Nor would his relatives be grateful. It was not unknown for terrible fights to break out in front of the graveyard gates between rival funeral processions rushing to bury their dead on the same day, each group of mourners determined that their late and dearly beloved one would not be the last to be buried. In October 1876, two men, who happened to be good friends, were simultaneously drowned in Tipperary, Ireland, when a cart they were driving fell into a river. The joint funeral turned into a general mêlée between rival groups of associates who believed that the second to be buried would be the servant of the other, and they would be punished.

While the origins of disease could be found in the supernatural, the symptoms could be treated with herbal and plant remedies. Many of these have found their way into the modern pharmacy. Willow bark was chewed to relieve pain, and its particular acid has been synthesized in aspirin. Foxgloves contain a poison – digitalis – that stimulates the heart. Many folk remedies are connected with the power believed to reside in certain animals, colours and numbers, and there are some your local doctor is unlikely to prescribe.

In Lincolnshire fried mice were reckoned excellent for whooping cough; in Yorkshire owls were used for the same purpose. Elsewhere, the first phlegm of the day was considered to be highly virtuous. In Demerara, earache was cured by boiling a cockroach in oil and stuffing it in the offending ear; and in Scotland warm cow dung was applied to open wounds, and fevers were cured by rubbing a live mole between one's hands until it expired. The poor mole was also much sought after in Sussex, where its paw was used to tackle toothache. The ashes of a dog were administered for rabies – hence the saying that you should take a hair of the dog that bit you. The cat has long been known to possess special powers, and in Scotland all sorts of complaints could be treated by cutting half the ear off your pet and letting the blood drip on the affected part. Slightly kinder was the idea of soothing rheumatism by putting a cat in your bed.

Electricity

Electricity, which has genuine and rather baffling therapeutic applications, was widely considered to be the new
marvel of surgery when it was first harnessed. All you
needed were two electrodes and a battery. Theories as to
how electricity could be used abounded in Victorian times,
and many claimed that mere exposure to an electrical field
could restore sexual prowess. Dr Julius Althaus, a Victorian
surgeon, wrote a little treatise on its application in cases of
impotence. His description of the recommended treatment may cause some discomfort in male readers. 'Spinal
impotency' was to be cured by inserting the anode of the
circuit up the penis while placing the cathode on the lower
back, in the lumbar region (this was before local anaesthetics). A current was then passed through which he
claimed would clear blockages, though as a consequence
the mucous membrane inside the penis tended to become
fused to the sizeable electrode inserted up it, which meant
that, left unattended, rigidity would never again be a
problem for the patient. Removal required reversal of the
current to free the flesh. 'If skilfully performed, this somewhat complicated proceeding is not unpleasant,' wrote
Althaus optimistically.

* * * * *

Toothache

Toothache was popularly believed to be caused by worms
breeding inside the jaw, and there are many pictures from
past centuries showing the fairground quack triumphantly
producing the tooth and a wriggling worm from inside the
mouth of the patient. Here's a 1607 version of some
eleventh century advice with a familiar ring:

> If in your teeth you hap to be tormented
> By meane some littles wormes therein do dwell
> Which pain (If need be tane) may be prevented

Bye keeping cleane your teeth when as you feed
Burne Frankincense (a gum not evil scented)
Put henbane into this and onyon seed
And with a tunnel to the roof that's hollow
Convey the smoke therof, and ease shall follow.

* * * * *

The Mineral Magnetizers

The mineral magnetizers, from the sixteenth century onwards, claimed that by harnessing the power of magnetism, diseases could be drawn out of the human body. In some cases, this doctrine was mixed with magical, alchemical and medical beliefs to create a hugely intricate and ritualized method of treatment. Paracelsus claimed that, using a magnet impregnated with 'mummy' – a derivative of corpses – and sprinkled with seeds which had a mythical congruity with the patient's affliction, he could draw the disease out of the body and into the seeds, which would then be planted. As the seeds sprouted into herbs, the disease would diminish. For an external growth or tumour, it was suggested that a powdered magnet be swallowed and a poultice of iron filings placed over the surface of the tumour. When the magnet, floating around inside the body, arrived underneath the tumour it would naturally be attracted to the iron filings outside the body and in attempting to suck them in, it would draw the sandwiched tumour back into the body. Any wound inflicted by a metallic weapon could be cured by magnetic principles: the sword simply had to be magnetized, after which it was dipped in the victim's blood and treated with ointment, as if it were the sufferer, while the patient was left to the whims of nature and whatever psychological effect this magic might have. One can imagine the increasingly gangrenous victim inquiring daily of his doctor how his weapon was progressing. This treatment, the 'Weapon-Salve', had many eminent believers.

Claudius Galen and the blood-letting disaster

One of the greatest figures in the entire history of medicine, and also one of the most remarkable quacks, was the physician Claudius Galen (c.130–210). Galen changed the face of medicine, largely for the better, but the harm he did, especially with one notable medical blunder, was incalculable. There have been other conspicuous medical big-heads, such as the celebrated German alchemist and physician Theophrastus Bombastus von Hohenheim (1493–1541), who called himself Paracelsus because he considered himself infinitely superior in knowledge and talent to the erudite and sophisticated Roman medical pundit Aulus Celsus. But even von Hohenheim could not hold a candle in self-admiration to Galen, whose many books – about 500 are attributed to him – are notable not only for the tremendous, if not always beneficial, influence they had on medicine for fifteen hundred years, but also for their almost unparalleled display of self-aggrandizement.

No one would try to deny that Galen was an extraordinarily gifted, learned and capable man. He was a Greek, born in AD 129 or 130 in Pergamum in north-west Asia Minor (modern Turkey), a city which at the time rivalled Alexandria in culture. His father, Aelius Nikon, was a prosperous architect and mathematician, who, when Galen was seventeen, had a dream (perhaps commoner with mothers than with fathers) which he interpreted as suggesting that his son should become a doctor. Galen had wanted to be a philosopher but was persuaded to change his mind. He was devoted to his father and made several affectionate references to him in his writings. His mother seems to have been a difficult woman from whom he probably derived some aspects of his character. Nikon was a generous man; no expense was spared in his son's education, and Galen studied at the University of Pergamum and then read medicine at the medical school (Aesculapion) there. Later, he went to Smyrna and Corinth to work under the best teachers, and to Alexandria where he spent much time in the great library poring over the works of Hippocrates, Aristotle and Plato.

At the age of twenty-eight Galen returned home, primed with knowledge and ready for anything. His first job was as a medical officer to a school of gladiators at Pergamum – an appointment made by the head priest at the Aesculapion. After about five years he decided that Pergamum did not offer him enough scope for his talents, so in the year AD 162, he went to Rome, where he called himself Claudius Galenus, and where he remained until he died in AD 201.

Some background information will help to explain Galen's extraordinary success as a doctor in Rome. The earliest Roman physicians had been slaves who could be bought and sold for the equivalent of a few hundred pounds – cheaper if they were eunuchs. Fortunately for Galen, Julius Caesar had, two hundred years before, granted freedom to all freeborn Greek physicians practicing anywhere in the Roman Empire. This raised the status of doctors considerably but did little to raise the standard of medical practice. Even so, some doctors did very well and a few became rich and famous. One former slave, Antonius Musa, for instance, accumulated a great fortune from private practice. Medical practice at the time was largely futile because it was not based on real knowledge. Although the Romans were more practical in their outlook than the Greeks – who always wanted to relate everything to philosophical theories – they had hardly begun to realize that the body and its diseases could be made the subject of practical study. Although they were splendid engineers and architects and were skilful in applying mechanical principles to such matters, it seemed to most of them that medical matters were still within the province of magic. Quacks and charlatans abounded in Rome, peddling stuff like crocodile droppings, camel's brains and turtle blood as sure-fire medicines.

No sooner did Galen arrive in Rome than he started quarrelling with his medical colleagues, missing no opportunity to point out how ignorant they were. The fact that, compared to him, they were ignorant hardly justified the bitter and self-laudatory tone he adopted. Galen loved medical argument, and because he had handled a human skeleton and done a few dissections of dead pigs, dogs and apes, and had a remarkable imagination, he always won. Human dissection was illegal during his lifetime, so he never had any real opportunity to find out whether the anatomy he claimed to know so well and described in such detail in his books was, in fact, correct. On the basis of a very little hard fact and an immense amount of guesswork, Galen soon built up a great edifice of medical lore which he claimed to be true. Since there was no one around who could question his dogmatic statements he got away with them. He began to give public lectures in anatomy and soon, to the annoyance of his colleagues, built up an enormous medical practice.

Galen loved to promote public arguments so that he could show off his knowledge. Soon – for people will often accept a notable figure at his own valuation – his opinion of himself was generally accepted and he was acknowledged to be on his own as the outstanding medical figure of the time. His reputation as a towering genius was established and there were few who dared to question his ideas. At the same time, inevitably, he excited the ill-will and envy of the other doctors. His response to criticism was an attack on his critics in language which, for violence and bitterness, became a byword and a topic of general amusement throughout the Roman Empire.

Naturally, Galen was in great demand, especially among the most celebrated and wealthy people of the time. The Emperor, Marcus Aurelius, was much troubled by upper abdominal discomfort and had been frightened by the dire prognostications of his doctors. Galen was summoned, carried out a careful examination, and announced that the trouble was nothing worse than indigestion. The Emperor was greatly impressed and Galen's reputation rose even further. Five years after he had settled in Rome, an epidemic of the plague broke out in that city and Galen, deciding that discretion was better than medical valour, made for home. He had other reasons for leaving Rome. His arguments with the other doctors, especially the members of the two predominant medical sects, the Methodists and the Erisistratists, and his methods of winning fame, made him so unpopular that Rome was becoming too hot to hold him.

He had hardly reached Pergamum, however, when a message reached him summoning him to attend on the Emperor who was, at the time, preparing to set out on a campaign to deal with some German tribes (Huns) who had dared to cross the Danube and were threatening northern Italy. Marcus was having a hard time of it, mainly because he was so short of money that he could hardly find the means to pay the additional two legions of soldiers he needed to meet the threat from the Huns. Things got so bad that he even had to auction some imperial property. Marcus wanted Galen to accompany him on the campaign, but Galen was not too keen on the idea of going to war, and told the Emperor that Aesculapius (the Roman god of medicine) had warned him in a dream not to go. Aurelius swallowed this story and excused him. In spite of this he appointed Galen as his personal physician and left him in Rome to look after the heir apparent, Commodus. This was the start of Galen's real success and he never looked back. For a quarter of a century he was physician to a succession of Roman emperors and prominent people and was undeniably medical top dog.

On Prognostics

In his book *On Prognostics* Galen wrote of himself: 'The Emperor never stops praising me. He has had experience of many money-grubbing, argumentative, conceited, envious and malignant doctors. He said of me: "Here is one physician who is never hide-bound by rules. Galen is the first of physicians and also of philosophers."' In *De Locis Affectis* he wrote: 'I completely won the admiration of the philosopher Glaucon by the diagnosis I made in the case of one of his friends. After this episode, Glaucon's confidence in me, and in my medical art, was unbounded.' In this book Galen recounts the episode in great detail so as to illustrate his own cleverness in diagnosis. Interestingly and impressively, he gives enough detail to show that he was able to associate liver disease with dysentery – what we now call amoebiasis – and was aware that liver problems of this kind can cause pain in the right shoulder. But it is only too clear from his account that his first concern was to impress the philosopher with his acumen.

In spite of his conceit and intolerance of criticism Galen was highly intelligent and, by any material or social standards, remarkably successful. Doctors with as much confidence as he had usually succeed. If the patient recovers, the doctor gets the credit; if he does not, the patient gets the blame. Galen was a keen observer with a remarkable memory and he became very skilful, from experience, at being able to predict the likely outcome of an illness (the prognosis) – an art which, although of no particular value to the patient, is very impressive to the ignorant. Characteristic of his arrogance is that he actually claimed that he had never been mistaken in a prognosis.

Whatever the reasons for his success, he enjoyed it in spite of professing a body of medical dogma that was remarkable for its errors and wrong-headedness. Although he knew something of the structure of the body, he was woefully ignorant of how it worked (its physiology), and he knew almost nothing of how to treat disease. His entire system was based on the extraordinary, and entirely imaginary, scheme – dreamed up by Hippocrates – that the body, like all nature, was composed of four elements – earth (dry), air (cold) fire (hot) and water (moist), and that everything that happened in the body, from illness to the manifestations of the personality, were governed by the four humours – blood, phlegm, black bile and yellow bile. These he elaborated into a vast and fantastic system that was to dominate medical thinking for centuries, to the exclusion of common sense, or, even, the immediate evidence of the senses.

Galen had something to say on every aspect of medicine, and was a great classifier. He was very strong on swellings (tumours), which he subdivided into *tumores secundum naturam* – all normal enlargements such as those of the female breasts at puberty and of the womb in pregnancy, *tumores supra naturam* – swellings from injury including the callus formation in healing bones, and *tumores praeter naturam* – in which group he lumped all cancers, cysts, inflammations, local oedemas and gangrene. So far as Galen was concerned, all ulcers were cancers and all cancers were caused by an excess of black bile. He insisted that his observations had proved that melancholic women were more prone to cancer than sanguine women and explained the prevalence of cancer of the breast and face (rodent ulcers) by asserting that these were the areas where the black bile thickened. Galen knew nothing about internal cancers or about the remote spread of cancers (metastases).

Mistaken theories

Many of his ideas were seriously mistaken. He taught that blood originated in the liver and was consumed in the other organs. He insisted that it passed through pores in the wall between the two sides of the heart and was mixed with air on the left side – an entirely imaginary process. He taught that the pulsation of the arteries served the same purpose as breathing, and he seemed to be confused as to whether or not arteries contained air – as the name implies and the Greek philosophers believed.

On the grounds that the action of the heart was involuntary, he denied that it was a muscle. He insisted, contrary to visible evidence, that the heart lay in the exact centre of the body. He believed that the brain generated a 'vital spirit' that passed through hollow nerves to the muscles, which it then activated. This idea was still universally credited as late as the end of the eighteenth century. He taught that phlegm originated in the brain rather than in the lining of the nose. He stated that cataracts were caused by a 'humour' from the brain that solidified behind the lens and insisted, against all evidence, that the lens occupied the centre of the eyeball. Galen repeatedly claimed respect, even reverence, for observed and demonstrable fact, but, in fact, his ideas were always dominated by his preconceived philosophical and mystical beliefs.

The most important consequence, for mankind, of the entirely imaginary humoural theory was the idea that disease could be cured by bleeding the patient – through 'blood-letting'. Galen insisted that the sanguine temperament was due to an excess of blood, so the prescription for anyone thought to be unduly 'plethoric', or to be suffering from any of the long list of 'sanguine' conditions, was, inevitably, bleeding. Of course, bleeding is an impressive activity. A vein is cut open and a pint or so of blood allowed to run into a bowl. If the removal of a pint or so of blood was not followed by a recovery, this was to be taken as a sign of the severity of the condition and as an indication of the need for further blood-letting.

This is a dreadful blunder, largely due to Galen's arrogant insistence on the truth of the humoural theory. In the centuries that followed, millions of people, many of whom desperately needed all the blood they could muster, were quite literally killed by doctors. Kings, Emperors, Popes, statesmen, gentry, common people were done away with. The more eminent the patient, the more likely he or she was to be bled to death. This professional slaughter, not only of upper class patients who could afford the attention of the physicians, but also of humbler gentry who were bled by barbers, continued until well into the eighteenth century.

Biography contains many graphic descriptions of the solemn deliberations of grave doctors, called in to treat famous personages, concluding that bleeding was indicated, and proceeding to the fatal process of exsanguination. Here is an edited account, taken from the novel *Gil Blas* by Le Sage (1668–1747) of the treatment by a Doctor Sangrado, which, although fictional, can be taken as typical of the activities of the Galen-inspired medicos of the time: 'For the first time in his life the Canon called in a physician. The distemper was fever; and it inflamed the gout. Doctor Sangrado was sent for; the Hippocrates of Valladolid. This learned forerunner of the undertaker had an aspect suited to his office: his words were weighed to a scruple; and his jargon sounded grand in the ears of the uninitiated. After studying my master's symptoms, he began with medical solemnity: the question here is, to remedy an obstructed perspiration. Sangrado then sent me for a surgeon of his own choosing, and took from him six good porringers (small pans) of blood, by way of a beginning. He then said to the surgeon: "Master Martin Onez, you will take as much more three hours hence, and tomorrow you will repeat the operation. It is a mere vulgar error that the blood is of any use in the system; the faster you draw it off the better. A patient has no more occasion for blood than a man in a trance; in both cases, life consists exclusively in pulsation and respiration." He then took his leave, telling me, with an air of confidence, that he would answer for the patient's life, if his system was fairly pursued. In less than two days the surgeon having bled him once more, the poor old man, quite exhausted, gave up the ghost under the lancet. Just as he was breathing his last, the physician made his appearance, and looked a little foolish, notwithstanding the universality of his deathbed experience. Yet far from imputing the accident to the bleeding, he walked off, affirming with intrepidity, that it was owing to their having been too lenient with the lancet.'

For many centuries, Galen was the therapeutic oracle whose opinions were engraved in stone and could not be wrong. His influence was so great that even when public readings from his texts were contradicted by the plain evidence of simultaneous dissections of the body, these discrepancies were ignored. Galen was, of necessity, correct, so the body in question must be abnormal. His writings were so powerful, so explanatory, so plausible and, above all, so authoritative, that they remained the standard texts until the sixteenth century, when they were forced to give way under the logical assaults of the great Flemish anatomist Andreas Vesalius (1514-64) and, later, William Harvey (1578–1657).

Even Vesalius, the foremost sixteenth-century anatomist and professor at the University of Padua, did not, at first, dare to challenge the writings of the great authority. But when artists, such as Leonardo da Vinci, who sketched accurately from human dissections and had no interest in medical dogma, showed that Galen was frequently mistaken, Vesalius took heart. In 1543 he published his masterpiece, *De fabrica corporis humani*, a beautifully illustrated text on human anatomy based on meticulous dissections and observations of dead bodies. This great work showed that many of Galen's ideas had been completely wrong.

Hahnemann and homoeopathy

The system of medical treatment or practice known as homoeopathy or homeopathy enjoys such a wide vogue at the present time and attracts so much money from the pockets of the uncritical that it demands close scrutiny. What is particularly interesting about the homoeopathy phenomenon is that it should persist in spite of the fact that its avowed basis is just about the most outrageous farrago of nonsense ever to be foisted upon the gullible public. If the basis of homoeopathy is true then the rest of medical science – indeed all science – is based on mistaken foundations and cannot be trusted.

The notion of homoeopathy was conceived by Christian Friedrich Hahnemann (1755–1843) – a complex character, the son of a Meissen porcelain painter. Hahnemann's father fell into poverty but the boy was so promising that his grammar-school education was continued by the generosity of his masters. Hahnemann worked hard and was granted free admission, as a poor scholar, to the College of Leipzig. While there, he supported himself by teaching French and Greek and by translating English texts into German. After completing the course at Leipzig, Hahnemann went to Vienna where he studied medicine and was appointed as personal physician and librarian to Baron von Bruckenthal at Hermanstadt. While there, Hahnemann became a Freemason and he retained his interest in Masonry for the rest of his life. His employment with the Baron allowed him to save enough money to complete his medical studies at Erlangen where he graduated MD in 1779.

Hahnemann now began to practice medicine. To his credit, it must be said that, in one of his appointments as physician to an asylum for the insane at Georgenthal, he followed the humanitarian practices of the great French psychiatric reformer Philippe Pinel and refused to adopt the standard and barbaric practices of physical restraint and punishment. So far, so good. Hahnemann then began to realize that the medical practices of the time were, on the whole, more likely to do harm than good and he soon became disenchanted with medicine. Among the practices that Hahnemann was perceptive and intelligent enough to see were foolish and dangerous was that of blood-letting. It was clear to him that to deprive a patient repeatedly of the vital fluid was to hasten his end. Indeed, Hahnemann was present at the death, from deliberate exsanguination, of more than one sick person who had the misfortune to be treated by his colleagues. So, rightly, he condemned this practice (see **Claudius Galen and the blood-letting disaster**). Hahnemann was also an advocate of good food, clean air and plenty of exercise.

Being extremely interested in chemistry he decided to give up medical practice and concentrate on chemistry and writing. He was a man of enormous energy and showed himself indefatigable, producing no less than fifty-eight volumes of original work in German and six volumes in Latin. In addition to this, he translated into German eleven medical works from English, five from French and one from Italian. Chemistry – which in those days was not clearly distinguished from pharmacology – went well and Hahnemann prospered. He was not, however, particularly scrupulous. He advertised and sold wares of some dubiousness. For instance, he sold plain borax at a high price under the name of *Pnoeum*, claiming that it was an original discovery of his own with great medicinal value. He also advertised a sure preventive for scarlet fever, keeping its nature secret until it was clear that, as a result of medical criticism, he would get nothing for it. He then admitted that it was belladonna – a drug that was liable to cause marked flushing of the skin and simulate to some extent the appearances of the scarlet fever rash. This episode clearly influenced his thinking, as will be seen. Hahnemann was not slow to turn his 'discoveries' to commercial advantage, by advertising his patent medicines. Only a year after abandoning the practice of medicine he wrote a book claiming that only the 'soluble mercury of Hahnemann' was any good in the treatment of venereal diseases. This work, entitled *Instructions for Surgeons on Venereal Diseases, with a New Preparation of Mercury* was an undisguised advertisement for his patent medication. In it he claimed that 'mercury removes all kinds of venereal mischief' – but only if it was of the Hahnemann brand.

Early doctrines

Unfortunately, as is often the case with men of such brilliance, he was also arrogant, big-headed, critical and argumentative. One thing he could not tolerate was any hint of criticism of his ideas or assertions. He asserted, for instance, that no substance dangerous to life could possibly enter the blood. This idea, so patently absurd, was, of course, challenged by his medical contemporaries. Hahnemann was a difficult man to argue with, partly because he was so irascible but also because he was a mass of self-contradictions. He was, apparently, wholly indifferent to inconsistency and, in his writings, often contradicts himself even in the same paragraph.

The doctrine of homoeopathy was first announced in Hufeland's *Journal of Practical Medicine* in 1796. Hufeland was an eminent physician who was attracted by Hahnemann's ideas but who was never able to accept them fully. The real exposition of homoeopathy was propounded at great length in Hahnemann's *Organon der Heilkunst* of 1810. To begin with, the *Organon* attracted very little interest but a year later Hahnemann succeeded in obtaining an appointment as a lecturer at the University of Leipzig and was able to promote his ideas. These were interrupted by the Napoleonic wars and it was not until 1813 that he was able to resume.

To his fury, he found that his ideas were opposed by the Professor of Medicine and condemned by other medical colleagues. At first, students used to attend his lectures for the fun of listening to his diatribes against the medical orthodoxy. But later these amusements palled and it became dangerous, in terms of medical politics to be seen there. So his audiences were soon reduced to a faithful handful of adherents.

Hahnemann based his system of medicine solely on symptoms and regarded any investigation into their cause as a waste of time. To Hahnemann, the symptoms were the disease and when these had been abolished the disease was cured. Anatomy, physiology, pathology and scientifically observed drug action, which were being patiently pursued by the best doctors of the time, he brushed aside as irrelevant. All diseases, he maintained, resulted either from conventional medical treatment or from one of three conditions – psora (the itch), syphilis or the skin disease sycosis. Most chronic diseases were caused by the itch being driven inwards. In order to cure disease, a remedy must be given which would substitute an effect similar to the symptoms but weaker. The principle was *similia similibus curantur*. To this end, Hahnemann studied the effects of many drugs on healthy people, selecting those which produced appropriate effects. Onions made the eyes water and the nose run; therefore onions were the very thing to treat the common cold. Arsenic produced the abdominal pain, vomiting and diarrhoea of dysentery; therefore arsenic was the very thing to treat dysentery. Atropine (belladonna) caused a hot, flushed skin, fever and hallucinations; therefore atropine was just what was needed for feverish illness such as scarlet fever. Obviously, there was no point in simply reproducing the symptoms of a disease and thus aggravating it. So these drugs must, he appreciated, be used in the smallest possible doses.

Mistaken assumptions

It was at this point that, intellectually, Hahnemann went completely off the rails. Observing that reducing doses of these mainly poisonous substances reduced their damaging effect, he made the extraordinary logical leap into the assertion that the benefit to be derived from these substances continued to increase as the dose was reduced. The simplest way to reduce the quantity was to dissolve the substance in water and then increase the dilution. Perhaps aware that this idea would probably be too much for anyone to swallow, he then formalized the notion into the remarkable theory of 'potentiation' by which, he claimed, medicines gained in strength by being diluted, so long as the dilution was accompanied by vigorous shaking or pounding. On this principle, he diluted his original tinctures to one fiftieth; these, in turn, to one fiftieth; and so on for thirty consecutive dilutions. This, the thirtieth consecutive dilution by fifty, was his favourite to which he ascribed the highest 'potentiality'. Serial dilution and shaking released a vital force which became stronger as the dilution increased – that is, as the amount of the original substance shrank to nothing. In the higher dilutions, Hahnemann claimed, this vital force was capable of being highly dangerous, so dangerous indeed that it might be too risky actually to drink the water. It would be sufficient just to sniff it carefully.

Hahnemann's enthusiasms were matched neither by his common sense nor his knowledge of arithmetic. If a solution is diluted as he prescribed, it is impossible that it should contain, except by accidental contamination, even a single molecule of the original substance. But he was not a man to be put off by such trifling detail. 'It is a therapeutic axiom,' he said, 'not to be refuted by all the experience in the world, that the best dose is always the smallest. He who does not walk on the same line with me is an apostate and a traitor.' In this he showed a characteristic common to many proponents of such systems – the belief a thing is true merely because they have said it. It seems clear, however, that Hahnemann secretly appreciated that he was talking and writing nonsense. The *Organon der Heilkunst*, in which he justifies homoeopathy, is written in such a metaphorical and hypothetical style as to be quite beyond anyone's power to understand. Had the whole thing – and the sixth and last edition of 1833 ran to 294 sections – been written in plain language it is probable that it would be seen to be absurd. Throughout the years Hahnemann frequently changed his mind on details so that successive editions of the *Organon* contained many contradictions. The books were written in numbered paragraphs with footnotes and the latter often became so voluminous that they displaced the main text. All this makes the study of Hahnemann's original writings on homoeopathy more than a little daunting. Perhaps this is not such a bad thing.

The hard-headed authorities in Leipzig, appalled by these ridiculous claims, barred him from practicing homoeopathy, but the French were more accommodating, and he settled in Paris where he eventually made a large fortune. He is said to have had an annual income of 200,000 francs.

Homoeopathy today
What is even more remarkable than Hahnemann's ideas is that,

in spite of all these manifest absurdities, the practice of homoeopathy should have persisted to this day. Modern practitioners of homoeopathy are, of course, unable to deny the simple mathematical facts about serial dilutions. They get round this by claiming that the real merit of homoeopathic dilution rests in the vigorous shaking that is given to each solution as it is diluted. This, they claim, confers some magic property on it. Because the word 'shaking' doesn't sound very impressive they prefer the term 'succussion' which means the same thing. Succussion can be hard work, so nowadays, it is usually done by machine. To some people, this ritual smacks of abracadabra. Insoluble substances, such as metals, are successively diluted with lactose (milk sugar) and are ground up in a mortar with a pestle. This grinding is said to be equivalent to succussion. It is worth mentioning that even the purest double-distilled water or the most refined lactose will, on the scale of dilution used in homoeopathy, contain molecules of many different substances including, very probably, those of the vital ingredient. This fact alone makes nonsense of the whole idea.

Notwithstanding that its principles run counter to everything science stands for, homoeopathy still enjoys a dubious respectability. In France, about a quarter of the doctors prescribe homoeopathic 'remedies'. The British public unthinkingly swallow millions of pounds worth of homoeopathy every year, to the satisfaction of the private pharmaceutical industry. There is a homoeopathic, if eclectic, hospital in London, and the NHS offers homoeopathic treatment, presumably on the principle that it is cheap and, of course, quite harmless.

This extraordinary state of affairs is hard to explain except on the basis that the general public simply do not know what homoeopathy is all about. But surely, this argument cannot apply to qualified medical practitioners who solemnly prescribe homoeopathic 'remedies'. How is it possible for people who purport to practice a scientific discipline to engage in treatment based on such ridiculous premises? The usual answer is that science has not yet advanced to the stage of being able to encompass homoeopathy, and that, in any case, homoeopathy works, so why knock it?

The plain truth is that homoeopathy does not work. People who take homoeopathic 'remedies' often feel better. This is especially so of those who are prescribed these things by practitioners who ask a lot of very detailed questions, some of which seem to have little relevance to the complaint, and then impressively work 'balanced formulations' to treat it. Sometimes the effect of this can seem remarkable, and both patient and doctor are confirmed in their view that 'there must be something in it'. It is not, of course, the infinitesimal dose of the homoeopathic 'remedy' that is producing this effect; it is the complex effect on the patient of the encouraging interaction with someone who seems to know what he or she is about and who apparently believes that he or she can do good.

This placebo effect is stronger than most people realize. As awareness of its power has grown, its definition has been extended. Formerly, a placebo was defined as a prescription given to satisfy a patient when there was no organic disorder but it was thought that a prescription was expected. It derives from the Latin verb *placere* meaning 'to appease or placate'. The term was also used to refer to a substance with no pharmacological effect, made to appear indistinguishable from a real drug, and used in clinical trials in comparison with the real thing, to determine how far the effects of the new drug under trial were genuinely due to its pharmacological action.

It is now recognized that the placebo effect is much more widespread than is implied in these limited definitions, and is present in almost all interactions between a therapist of any kind, real or claimed, and a person in the role of patient. It even operates between lay people when one claims medical knowledge, and comments, encouragingly or optimistically, on another's condition. The placebo effect operates on the brain and can modify the symptoms of many conditions, sometimes more profoundly than can active drugs.

This is especially true of pain, in which the psychological component is often as important as the sensory in determining the significance of the pain to the individual. Opiate drugs, including the natural opiates, the endorphins, do not necessarily remove the pain, but they may so modify the attitude to it that the affected person ceases to be concerned about it. It is not widely known, but highly significant, that people receiving 'pain-killing' tablets of milk sugar, which they believe to be a strong pain-killing drug, actually show raised levels of endorphins in their blood.

The implications of all this are profound, especially in relation to the great range of unorthodox 'therapies' including homoeopathy. The placebo effect of this kind of practice may be very great and the sufferer may derive remarkable, although usually transient, relief. It is, however, important to appreciate the difference between subjective effects of this kind and a genuine cure of a disorder. Certainly, 'feeling better' is no basis for scientific validation of the method.

Critics of homoeopathy

The great American writer and physician Oliver Wendell Holmes (1809–94) put the matter a little differently in his essay, *Homeopathy and its Kindred Delusions*: 'So long as the body is affected through the mind, no audacious device, even of the most manifestly dishonest character, can fail of producing occasional good to those who yield it an implicit or even a partial faith. Homeopathy is a mingled mass of perverse ingenuity, of tinsel erudition, of imbecile credulity, and of artful misrepresentation, too often mingled in practice with heartless and shameless imposition.'

Perhaps the most important reason why homoeopathy should be regarded as one of the greatest medical blunders of all time is this: science has had a very hard time, throughout recent centuries, in dragging mankind up out of the quagmire of superstition, witchcraft and magic. We may laughingly suppose that these are all things of the dark ages, but there is no reason to do so. Human nature has not changed in the 300 years since we held beliefs that, we felt, entirely justified us in tying old women to stakes and burning them to death. There is no particular reason for us to be complacent; other civilizations have descended from enlightenment to barbarity. So there are sound reasons for challenging any system that ignores or attacks the principles on which our present level of civilization depends. Homoeopathy is not, of course, the only activity that substitutes magic and superstition for reliable truth; many branches of alternative medicine and much of the Mind and Spirit Movement also do so.

No doubt many aspects of contemporary scientific medicine can legitimately be criticized, but at least it can claim to be based on thoroughly tested and rational facts. These facts are derived from observation and carefully-controlled experiment and they are so thoroughly tested that every day millions of people's lives depend on their being correct. When a disorder is found and its details clearly understood, scientific medicine responds by taking rational steps to oppose its cause. The scientific doctor is not concerned with trying to remove symptoms; he or she is concerned to discover the cause of the trouble and, if possible, to remove it so that the whole disorder, including the symptoms, is removed. Homoeopathy is based on magic. It has no rational basis and its assertions not only have nothing to do with science – they are actually anti-scientific.

Perhaps the public perception of the scientific doctor is at the root of the problem. Scientific doctors are often perceived as being cold, technologically-oriented, lacking in humanity and preoccupied with prescribing powerful drugs with dangerous side effects. No doubt there are such doctors, but they are few and far between. Good doctors are always concerned with human factors and are holistic in their approach to patients. The reason they often seem short on human qualities is much more often that they are so busy that they simply cannot afford the time to give their patients what they need – a little warmth and sympathy.

The water cure

Vincenz Priessnitz, who was born in 1799, was an uneducated Silesian peasant farm labourer but a person of remarkable character and abilities. When he was a young man he was kicked in the face by a horse, knocked to the ground and run over by a cart. Vincenz lay in agony and a surgeon was called. He found that two of his ribs were broken, shook his head gravely and announced that Vincenz would never work again.

The young man declined to accept this prognosis, however.

Having been taken indoors, he rested for a time then decided to cure himself. By pressing his body against the edge of a table and taking very deep breaths, he was actually able to set the fractured ribs. Immediately he was relieved of much of the pain in his chest. Now able to move gingerly he soaked some cloths in water and pressed them to the injured areas of his body. He then remained still to allow the rib fractures to heal.

For a week Vincenz lay quietly, moving only to renew the wet cloths and eating nothing. He did, however, drink copious quantities of water. At the end of a week he was up and about, almost free from pain. Within a few months he was fully recovered and able to undertake strenuous work. This experience convinced him that pure water, used both externally and internally, could cure any disorder of the body. But Vincenz was not content to leave the matter at that. If water could cure, how did it do so?

Gradually, he evolved an impressive theory of disease in which all bodily upsets, except those caused by physical injury, were the result of the accumulation in the body of substances he called 'bad juices'. These poisonous juices arose as a result of various influences such as unsatisfactory food, bad air, insufficient exercise, worry, and, in particular, failure of free perspiration. Bad juices could have a general effect and produce general disease, such as a fever, or they could concentrate in one area to cause a local disorder, such as gout.

Clearly, if the body could be relieved of the bad juices, recovery from disease would follow. It was equally obvious to Vincenz that the one way to get rid of the bad juices was by the use of pure water and by the encouragement of free perspiration. Vincenz's ideas seemed eminently sensible to his contemporaries and many patients came to him for advice and treatment. He was so successful as a healer that, eventually, in 1829, he set up a treatment spa at Gräfenberg. This enterprise flourished remarkably and by 1840 he was treating as many as 1,400 patients every year. His fame spread and he included among his clientele many members of the European royal families.

At the Gräfenberg Spa Vincenz expected his patients to drink at least twelve glasses of water each day. In addition, they were wrapped up in blankets on a feather bed with only the face exposed and, while so covered, had to drink a glass of water every half hour to promote sweating. Turning a bright pink colour was an excellent sign of the removal of bad juices and when this happened patients were immersed in cold water for several minutes. Occasionally water was also given as an enema.

Because he had no medical qualifications Vincenz aroused the suspicion and resentment of the Austrian medical establishment. So a committee was set up to investigate his spa. Happily, because he used neither drugs nor surgery, the inspectors could find nothing to complain about. Indeed, the chief inspector, after a visit to Gräfenberg, found that many patients were improved by the treatment and none were harmed. His report did much to encourage patients.

Vincenz had certainly started something. The official report, together with the support and recommendation of his many aristocratic patients, soon led to the spread of the water cure. Before long nearly fifty such establishments were set up in most countries in Europe and in Russia and about two hundred were set up in the Americas. Hydropathy, as it was called, became all the vogue and hydropathic medical schools sprang up everywhere.

There were considerable merits in Vincenz's system, the principal one being that, unlike other systems of doctoring, it did no harm. The method allowed the body's natural healing powers to operate unchecked without interference from such damaging practices as blood-letting or the administration of poisonous drugs. It also encouraged cleanliness of the skin and a reduced dietary intake and increased urinary output. If you drink as much water as Vincenz prescribed, you will find it impossible to eat very much. So, although the system was based on a theory with no scientific foundation it was, for its time, admirable.

As medical science advanced, especially with the discovery by Louis Pasteur of bacteria in the early 1860s, the true cause of many diseases became apparent and hydropathy gradually faded. Nevertheless, during the heyday of his system, Vincenz Priessnitz had done more for suffering humanity than most doctors of his time.

The X-ray cure

The index for the *British Medical Journal* for 1896 contains no entries under X. This is because it was not until late one November afternoon in 1895 that the German professor Wilhelm Conrad Röntgen (1845–1923) first observed the phenomenon that was to become so important in medicine. Röntgen was experimenting with 'cathode rays' using a glass tube with metal electrodes sealed into both ends and most of the air sucked out. He was working in the dark and had connected the electrodes in the tube to a high-voltage induction coil. When he switched on the current he happened to notice a faint greenish glow coming from something on a bench some distance away. When he switched off, the glow disappeared. He switched on and off several times and each time the glow appeared and went.

This seemingly trifling observation was to revolutionize medical diagnosis and was to win Röntgen the Nobel Prize for physics in 1901. It was also to lead to a serious medical blunder. Cathode rays are streams of electrons. We now know that if electrons are accelerated by a high voltage and caused to strike a piece of material such as metal or glass, electrons will be knocked out of the inner orbits of the atoms of the material. When this happens, outer electrons of higher potential energy than those displaced fall inwards to take their place, releasing energy in the form of electromagnetic waves of shorter wavelength than ultraviolet light. These are the X-rays, so called by Röntgen because he had no idea what they were.

Nor, of course, did Röntgen have the least idea of the atomic mechanism by which the new ray was produced. After observing the glow, Röntgen lit a match and found that it was coming from a small sheet of cardboard that had been coated with a chemical that was known to glow when struck by various kinds of ray. This new ray, however, was invisible. He was amazed at his discovery but soon became dumbfounded when he noted that the card would still glow even if a sheet of thick black paper were interposed between it and the tube.

This set him to experimenting furiously and in the days that followed he found that the new ray would pass through wood, through thin sheets of metal and, to his further amazement, his own hand. When he tried this, he found that he could make out on the coated card, the outline shadow of his fingers and, within these, the denser shadow of his fingers. As he moved his fingers, he watched the bones moving. Röntgen was a keen photographer and it was not long before he had substituted a wrapped photographic plate for the fluorescing screen. With this, he made a historic and permanent photograph of the bones of his wife's hand, on which her wedding ring is clearly visible.

Röntgen immediately announced his discovery and the important implications for medicine and industry. Immediately, manufacturers saw the importance of getting into the act and X-ray apparatus began to be mass-produced. X-rays were also of considerable novelty value and were widely demonstrated in department stores and elsewhere. Shoe shops installed X-ray equipment so that customers could see that their shoes fitted properly. People using this equipment constantly soon noticed, however, that they could not do so with complete impunity. Some of these demonstrators began to notice that parts exposed to the rays developed a kind of painful sunburn. Their fingernails stopped growing and in some cases eyelashes and head hair fell out.

Röntgen was a true scientist and continued to investigate the properties of X-rays and to publish papers on the subject. Although he was, of course, well aware of the commercial value of his discovery he made no attempt to patent it or otherwise to benefit financially from it. Others were less scrupulous. Whenever a new principle becomes fashionable someone can be relied on to suggest that it must have medical value as a form of treatment. This happened with the development of chemistry and when it was discovered that electricity could be generated. Exactly the same thing happened with X-rays.

The new phenomenon was taken up enthusiastically by many doctors and applied indifferently for the treatment of all sorts of conditions. There was no real excuse for the reckless way in which X-rays were used. There was plenty of evidence that these rays were damaging to human tissue. Long exposures were necessary for chest and abdominal pictures and people who lay under X-rays for several sessions of 20 minutes or so would suffer 'sunburn' that developed into large and intensely painful ulcers. Some of the most distinguished and careful doctors warned against them. As early as 1896, the great English surgeon and pioneer of antiseptic surgery Sir Joseph Lister (1827–1912) described the effects of overdosage. Lister did, however, suggest that X-rays might produce 'salutary stimulation' and this may have encouraged the less scrupulous of his colleagues. None of these doctors had any idea of the real dangers to which they were exposing their patients – and often their own bodies.

Dermatologists were particularly keen on X-rays and tried them on their patients for practically every form of skin disease. Some seemed to get better and so encouraged further use of the method; others did not. All of these patients later suffered ill effects ranging from the annoying to the fatal. Adolescents with acne were extensively irradiated. Children with fungus infection of the scalp were given X-rays until all their hair fell out. Birthmarks were treated with X-rays. Tennis elbow and other forms of bursitis; shoulder pain, often inadequately diagnosed; adenoids; Eustachian catarrh; shingles; enlarged thymus in infants; mumps; sterility from ovarian dysfunction; arthritis of the neck; ankylosing spondylitis (poker back from fusion of the vertebrae); carbuncles of the neck; keloid scars; and many other conditions were, as recently as 1960, routinely treated by X-rays. These treatments were actually and solemnly advised in medical textbooks of all kinds.

In the Röntgen Institute, St George's Hospital, Hamburg, is a tall standing stone plaque – a monument on which are engraved the names of scores of early workers with X-rays who suffered and died as a result of their practice and their research. These names are a mere handful by comparison with the thousands of patients who suffered as a result of useless and dangerous treatments with X-rays. Today, most doctors are unaware of the extent of this terrible blunder. Older physicians, aware that no present-day doctor would dream of using such treatments, tend to forget, or repress the memory, of how confidently they would once, as young professionals, have recommended them.

The origins of radiotherapy

It was not long after Röntgen's discovery that it was found that certain forms of cancer would seemingly melt away under the influence of X-rays. This was the beginning of the now very important speciality of radiotherapy. Many cures were claimed when, in fact, the tumours were merely reduced in size and soon recurred. Doctors were aware that cancers were masses of living cells similar to those of the rest of the body. If these cells could be killed by X-rays, it should have been apparent, and obviously was to many, that normal cells could also be killed. What was not apparent was that X-rays in much smaller doses than were required to kill cancers could actually cause cancers. Nowadays we are all familiar with the effects of radiation on DNA and are all acutely aware of the dangers of radiation. The early medical pioneers of X-ray work had none of the benefits of this knowledge and the results were, of course, disastrous. Thousands of people developed chronic skin ulcers, skin cancers, leukaemia, cessation of red cell production (aplastic anaemia) and genetic damage to their offspring.

Today, we worry about doses of X-radiation which are a small fraction of the doses casually given to patients, often for trivial conditions, earlier this century.

Röntgen postscript
In Röntgen's apparatus, the X-rays were actually produced by the atoms of the glass of the tube. Modern X-ray tubes are slightly different from, and very much more efficient than, Röntgen's original version. The electrons are obtained from a strong, electrically heated filament, as in a modern TV tube. This is called the cathode. Electrons are negatively charged and are attracted across the tube to a block of tungsten to which a high positive voltage is applied. This is the anode. The tungsten anode is angled so that the X-rays are passed out of the side of the tube. It is also cooled by circulating water. TV tubes also use a high positive voltage to attract electrons to the screen, but fortunately for all of us, the electron beam is swung about rapidly all over the face of the tube and merely cause the phosphors on the inside of the tube face to glow. Very little in the way of X-rays are emitted by modern TV receivers.

The blue glass cure-all

In 1876 General Augustus J. Pleasonton, a Union officer in the American civil war, published a remarkable book entitled *The Influence of the Blue Ray of the Sunlight and of the Blue Colour of the Sky*. The title page continued with the legend 'IN DEVELOPING ANIMAL AND VEGETABLE LIFE; IN ARRESTING DISEASE, AND IN RESTORING HEALTH IN

ACUTE AND CHRONIC DISORDERS TO HUMAN AND DOMESTIC ANIMALS'. The book contained full details of the experiments with blue glass which the distinguished General had been conducting since 1861. Blue light, it seemed, was a panacea for almost all diseases.

The work was an immediate success, was widely read and its claims widely confirmed. Testimonials poured in from people famous and otherwise. State governors, well-known authors, ministers of religion, actors and others wrote to confirm the wonderful therapeutic power of blue glass. All over the country people were knocking out plain glass from one of their windows and substituting a blue pane. A window in the south side of the house was best, and the results could be magical. People with smallpox were instantly cured. Blue light was a sure cure for insanity – witness the reports in *The American Journal of Mental Science* and *The British Journal of Psychological Medicine*. One man whose leg was about to be amputated for gangrene fitted a blue pane and sent the surgeon packing. Many blind people were restored to sight.

Blue light was invaluable for animals as well as humans. One of the most remarkable cures was reported by a farmer who had had his best boar castrated and had then regretted it. So he locked up the boar in a henhouse and fitted a pane of blue glass. The results were nothing short of miraculous. Within a period actually less than the usual gestation time, the farmer's finest sow brought forth a litter of unprecedented size and quality. This was clearly a medical advance of the first importance. The newspapers were full of the sensation. The learned journals took it up. The enthusiasm was enormous.

Sadly and unaccountably, blue glass was never incorporated into the body of orthodox medical practice. The reasons for this extraordinary omission have never been satisfactorily explained.

The focal sepsis affair

There is an unpleasant eye condition in which the iris – the colored part of the eye – and the ring-shaped muscle around the iris root become inflamed. The iris has a round hole in its center called the pupil, and tiny muscles in the iris control the size of the pupil. In bright light the pupil becomes small and in dim light it enlarges. The ring muscle that surrounds the iris is called the ciliary body and is responsible for the focusing of the eye. Inflammation of these two parts of the eye is called iridocyclitis or uveitis.

This inflammation causes a dull aching pain in the eye and both the iris and the ciliary body become swollen. As a result the pupil becomes small even in the dark. Iris inflammation also causes it to give off a sticky discharge so that the water inside the eye – the aqueous humour – becomes milky and vision becomes misty. The sticky iris commonly becomes glued to the internal lens immediately behind it and this can cause an obstruction in the outflow of the water that is constantly being produced inside the eye. The inflammation of the ciliary body prevents focusing and is reflected in quite severe redness of the white of the eye around the margin of the cornea.

As well as being smaller than the other pupil, the affected pupil is often of irregular outline. The iris may appear to be of a slightly different colour from the healthy one. Treatment is urgent because if the adhesions to the front surface of the crystalline lens become firm and the outflow of aqueous humour is blocked, the pressure in the eye will rise and permanent damage will result. This rise in internal pressure is called acute glaucoma and must at all costs be avoided.

So long as the condition is not mistaken for simple conjunctivitis – which is nearly always caused by infection – effective treatment to widen the pupil – usually with atropine – and damp down the inflammation – usually with steroid eye drops – will control the situation.

For years, doctors simply had no idea of the cause of iridocyclitis. It had been known for many years that the condition often occurred in people suffering from syphilis or tuberculosis and it is still a routine procedure in cases of the condition to do a VDRL test for syphilis, a chest X-ray and other tests for TB, and a check for diabetes. Various other investigations are also usually carried out but, today, in the great majority of cases, no additional disease is found to which the eye problem can be attributed. The mere presence of other disease, of course, does not imply that this is the cause of the iridocyclitis.

A situation such as this is ripe for 'explanatory' hypotheses and these were not long in coming. From the late nineteenth century until well into the 1970s many doctors subscribed to the 'focal sepsis' hypothesis. Indeed, for most of the first half of the twentieth century, this was generally accepted as the common cause of those cases of iridocyclitis in which no other explanation was forthcoming. This idea amounted to no more than the notion that iridocyclitis was actually a recurrent infection and that the source of the germs was some hidden focus of infection somewhere in the body. Germs from this infected site, or possibly, toxins from germs, were thought to be released into the bloodstream and carried to the eye or eyes to bring about the inflammation.

These sites of focal infection were thought to be most likely to occur in the teeth, tonsils, nasal sinuses, prostate gland (in men), urinary tract or bowel. They might, of course, be elsewhere. As a result of this imaginary notion which is now dismissed by the experts, thousands of people had a total dental clearance, had their normal tonsils removed, their normal sinuses washed out, underwent unnecessary appendicectomy, suffered high colonic irrigation, or were exposed to a range of other pointless treatments. It is hardly necessary to state that none of these people enjoyed any ocular benefit from any of these procedures.

Today, because of the enormous advances in understanding of the immune system that occurred largely as a result of the AIDS epidemic, it seems clear that most cases of iridocyclitis are caused by what is known as an autoimmune process. This means that the immune system, for various reasons, chooses to recognize certain parts of the body as being foreign tissue and attacks them. All body cells carry surface markings by which the cells of the immune system can recognize them as 'self'. Foreign invaders such as germs or transplanted tissue carry different surface markings and are recognized as 'foreign'. Antibodies are then produced that attach to the invaders enabling them to be attacked and, if possible, destroyed. Although the full details of the process are still not understood, there is good evidence that this is the kind of process that produced the recurrent inflammation of the iris and ciliary body known as iridocyclitis.

Aldous Huxley
One of the most famous sufferers from iridocyclitis was the novelist and philosophical writer Aldous Huxley (1894–1963).

Huxley suffered recurrent attacks, often affecting both eyes and was, intermittently, so seriously disabled by poor vision that his career was affected. The trouble started in 1910 when he was sixteen at Eton. His cousin Gervas was ready to apportion blame and confidently wrote: 'When run down after influenza and out on a field day with the Eton ORC, a streptococcus infection from dust attacked his eyes. Had penicillin been discovered it would, no doubt, have cleared the whole thing up in a short time, but as it was, the Eton authorities neglected his condition and he had almost completely lost the sight of both eyes before his father was informed and brought him to London to see specialists.' This idea of the causation of the disorder was nonsense, but it is true that any delay in seeking specialist attention could have been very serious. As it was, Huxley's vision was reduced to bare perception of light in one eye and about one tenth of normal in the other. He showed extraordinary courage and immediately started to learn Braille. Fortunately, his vision eventually improved enough to enable him to read.

Perhaps influenced by his brother Julian, he had intended to study biology, but instead turned to English. Later, the disease caused him to move to the more equable climate of California where he became involved in the drug culture. Huxley was a man of extraordinary intellect who was interested in everything, but did not always have the detachment necessary for a properly scientific approach to the problems of his eye disorder. Iridocyclitis is a condition of frequent recurrences and remissions and Huxley became convinced that various unorthodox treatments he adopted were the cause of his improvements. In particular, he was seduced by the fatuous writings of the American quack Dr W.H. Bates. Huxley was not the only one to be taken in by this gentleman's plausible arguments. Bates' book *Perfect Sight Without Glasses* (New York, 1920) has been a long-term best-seller and has gone into over 30 editions. It is still on sale today. Huxley's own book on the subject, *The Art of Seeing* (Chatto & Windus, 1943) is a much better book and concentrates on the psychology of perception and on trying to improve it in various ways. Nevertheless, it is full of medical misconceptions, purely imaginary ideas and some distinctly dubious practices. Huxley, for instance, advocates looking briefly at the sun. This can be dangerous and can actually destroy the cones in the central and most essential parts of the two retinas. He was deeply impressed by Bates' method of 'palming' – a procedure in which the eyes are pressed with the flat of the palms. He did not, apparently understand that this can temporarily alter the curvature of the corneas and shorten the axial length of the eyes, both of which could briefly improve vision. Nor did he seemingly appreciate that his advice to 'exercise' the eyes by reading very small print would produce the promised improvement only if associated, as he also dictates, with very bright light on the paper. Bright light, of course, will 'stop down' the pupil so much, and so greatly increase the depth of focus, that it may allow reading without glasses by people who normally need them. Every presbyope is familiar with the importance of a good light for easy reading.

It is an extraordinary commentary on the power of suggestion that a man of his intellectual capacity who must have been much more aware than most of the common *post hoc ergo propter hoc* (after this, therefore, because of this) logical fallacy, was, nevertheless, taken in by it. In the less affected eye, Huxley had a heavy deposit of inflammatory cells on the centre of the inner surface of his cornea. This so fogged out his vision that the eye was of little use. He could improve the vision by keeping the pupil widened with atropine drops so as partly to clear the opaque patch. As is characteristic of these corneal deposits, this patch, washed continuously by circulating aqueous humour, gradually absorbed. It is possible that Huxley's regular 'palming' by repeatedly indenting his corneas, may have helped to disperse these deposits.

None of this should be taken to detract in any way from Huxley's merits as a novelist or philosophical thinker. And it is only fair to comment that his blunders, in this context, sink into insignificance when compared with those of the doctors.

The bed rest blunder

There is a conventional idea that if you are sick, you should go to bed. Certainly if you are acutely ill, fevered or weakened by disease it is a comfort to rest in a well-made bed, and no one would deny that this is desirable. But doctors now recognize that it is wrong to infer from this that everyone suffering from any disease whatsoever should automatically be confined to bed. A fuller understanding of bodily processes and of the way the body responds to activity has led, in recent years, to a fairly radical change of ideas about the importance of bed rest for the sick. Enforced bed rest, except for the reasons mentioned above, is now recognized as having been a major medical blunder for which many unfortunate patients have suffered dearly.

In the past it has been assumed that bed rest *per se* has some kind of healing properties. Doctors have rationalized that, by resting in bed, the patient has been able to devote all his or her 'strength' to 'fighting' the illness. This is all nonsense. Another reason for bed restriction has sometimes been the will of autocratic nursing Sisters more concerned with their own administrative convenience and with the exercise of power than with any considerations of its advantage to the patient. Formerly, any person who became a hospital patient was expected to conform to a role in which he or she was wholly subservient to the will of the medical and nursing staff. Regrettably, even in a caring profession such as medicine, power corrupts and some people are more easily corrupted by it than others. So the regimented ward, with patients lying straight and all neatly covered up by sheets, blankets and bedcovers, was too often assumed to be normal and right. This pattern may have helped to formalize the convention. Unfortunately, many of the patients who were forced to conform in this way would have been very much better off strolling about the hospital grounds or playing table tennis. But that would have been untidy and perhaps some patients would not have been immediately to hand come enema time.

Happily, modern ward Sisters are much more humane and, in addition, doctors now know that bed rest often does more harm than good. Prolonged rest is, in itself, surprisingly harmful. A person who spends an unnecessary month in bed, and is then allowed to get up, will take at least a month to recover fully from the damage done by the period spent in bed. This may seem a surprising statement but there is a good physiological reason for it. At any age, the body responds to the physical demands made upon it, and does so exactly to the extent that these demands are made. We are all familiar with the way athletes, by training, increase their physical ability or body builders, by muscular work, get to look quite ridiculous. This same process applies to everyone, young or old. The body's capacity for work will, within limits, adapt to the demands made upon it. Thus, enforced bed rest, unless clinically necessary, is damaging and often leads to a notable decline in fitness.

The structure of muscles

One reason people find all this hard to believe is because they have a quite unreal conception of muscles and bones. This idea is derived from the butcher's shop where muscle (meat) is coagulated and bones dried. Living muscles are not solid, fixed structures as most people seem to think. They are more like fluid jellies, and their constituents – mainly amino acids – are flowing in and out of them, and of the blood, all the time. If muscles are used, their fibres (cells) will become more bulky; if they are not used the fibres will atrophy. Much the same goes for bones. These are different from dried bones in a museum. Calcium, phosphorus and the protein building-blocks (amino acids) are flowing in and out all the time. If the bones need greater strength, the net inflow of these constituents will be greater; if they are not exposed to physical stress, the outflow will be greater. Joints can readily stiffen and will do so if not put through their normal range of movement. If the full range of movement is not regularly used, the range will soon become narrowed. One of the signs of ageing is the restriction of joint movement and this is entirely due to reduced activity. A joint that is not moved at all for weeks or months may become permanently fixed and solid.

Rest is thus damaging to muscle power, to agility, to joint movement and to the strength of the bones. Young people can usually get back to their former state after a period of enforced rest, but elderly people confined to bed may never recover their former vitality. Muscles weaken and lose bulk; bones lose calcium and lose their basic protein bulk. This is called osteoporosis and it makes bones more liable to fracture. Once it has occurred, it is very hard to reverse, especially in older people.

Another bad effect of prolonged rest is the development of pressure sores (bed sores). These occur at points where the weight of the body is taken on bony protrusions, and mainly affect the buttocks, the heels, the elbows and the back of the head. Bedsores may be very large and the ulceration may progress to complete local loss of skin with exposure of the underlying tendons or bone.

Unduly prolonged bed rest also results in a drop in the efficiency of the heart, and a markedly increased tendency for clotting to occur in the large veins of the legs (deep vein thrombosis). The latter is especially common after surgical operations in the elderly. Vein thrombosis commonly leads to the formation, within the veins, of a loose, gelatinous and everlengthening snake-like blood clot which, initially attached at one end, may break loose and be carried up to the heart whence it is pumped to the lungs to cause a highly dangerous obstruction to one of the main arteries. This is called pulmonary embolism and is often fatal. It is a common cause of death in inactive older people, especially those in hospital or confined to bed at home.

Nowadays, doctors are acutely conscious of the need to avoid this medical blunder and will sometimes seem to be unkind in their anxiety to get patients out of bed. But they know very well, often from bitter personal experience, that it is all too easy to kill by kindness.

Chapter Two

Sexual healing

Circumcision

The term 'circumcision' literally means 'cutting around'. In reality it means the removal of the male foreskin, whether done surgically for medical reasons or ritually for other reasons. The history of this extraordinary practice goes back into the mists of time and it has been an important part of the ritual of many different cultures. The earliest known use of circumcision was in Egypt as long ago as 2300 BC. The purpose, then, is thought to have been the marking of slaves. It is routinely carried out in most parts of Africa, south-east Asia, Australia and the Pacific Islands. It is routine with Orthodox Muslims to whom it symbolises spiritual purification, and is performed either in infancy or prior to marriage. Gurkha soldiers carry their removed foreskins in a little brass box suspended from a string slung round their necks.

Male Jewish babies are circumcised on the eighth day after birth in accordance with Abraham's covenant with God, and all males converted to Judaism have to submit to circumcision. The practice is so well ingrained that many Jews who have abandoned all other religious beliefs and practices will still opt for circumcision for their children. To the orthodox, the procedure is of the highest religious significance.

Opinions on the medical and social merits of circumcision have been hotly debated for decades, and the facts have been somewhat distorted by argument and prejudice – to say nothing of ignorance of a few basic physiological facts. During development, the foreskin is initially attached to the bulb (glans) of the penis and this attachment, in the form of a few tissue strands normally persists during the early months of life. For this reason, it is perfectly normal not to be able to pull the foreskin back. Failure to do so is certainly not grounds for circumcision.

In babies and little boys the opening at the tip of the foreskin is normally quite small, but will stretch in time. If, however, the opening is no more than a pin-point and is so small that the foreskin balloons out when the baby is urinating, circumcision is justified. This condition of an abnormally small opening is called *phimosis* and can lead to later trouble. Back-pressure of urine is to be avoided as it can cause urinary tract infection and kidney damage. Circumcision eliminates this risk, but the risk exists only if the outlet is extremely narrow. This is uncommon. A report in the *American Journal of Pediatrics* that uncircumcised boys were ten times more likely to develop urinary tract infections than the circumcised was widely reported in the public press and has probably fortified the American public in its apparent conviction that nature has somehow got the human anatomy wrong.

It is a great mistake to get obsessive about a tight foreskin, as some mothers do, and to keep trying to pull it back. But occasional attempts at gentle retraction will do little boys no harm and will help to stretch the skin. Later, it is important to be able to pull the foreskin right back so that the creamy, cheesy-looking, and nasty-smelling material, smegma, which collects under it, can be washed away every day. Full retraction is achieved gradually and may take months. It should certainly be possible by late adolescence. If not, circumcision should be considered.

Smegma has excited a good deal of interest among doctors and there have been suggestions that it can cause cancer of the penis and of the cervix in women. These ideas have been cited as justification for circumcision. They are, however, based on very dubious evidence. Horse smegma, repeatedly rubbed into the shaven skin of mice was shown to be capable of causing a form of skin cancer. Like most good stories, this one has been widely quoted in medical circles and widely believed by lay people. One perceptive critic remarked that this was rather hard on the mice and that he would have been much more impressed if the researchers had been able to produce skin cancer in horses by rubbing in mouse smegma.

Another circumstance cited as 'proof' that smegma was carcinogenic, was the well-established fact that married Jewish women had a much lower incidence of cervical cancer than married Gentile women. This seemed impressive at first until it was shown that the difference could be accounted for on the basis of the virus that has been implicated in the causation of cervical cancer – the human *papillomavirus*. This virus is known to be sexually transmitted and accounts for the higher incidence of cervical cancer in sexually promiscuous women. Jewish sexual laws and family traditions, the difference in the number of sexual partners, the avoidance of sex during menstrual periods, and other factors, readily explain the reduced incidence in Jewish women.

So far as cancer of the penis is concerned, it is true that this is almost unknown in circumcised men. But there is a good reason for this. Penile cancer nearly always starts on the inner surface of the foreskin, in men with poor standards of personal hygiene. Long-persisting irritation from accumulated smegma could be a factor. But it is worth noting that cancer of the penis is also almost unknown in uncircumcised men – only about one hundred cases occur each year in Britain – so the argument is a little forced.

The latest American attack on the foreskin comes in the form of a suggestion, in a letter in the *New England Journal of Medicine*, that uncircumcised men are more likely to acquire AIDS than the circumcised. The author bemoans the declining rate of circumcision and hints that the policy may be regretted.

One can probably get closest to the truth of the matter by looking at the figures for circumcision in societies in which surgery has to be paid for, and comparing them with the figures in societies where surgery is free. For years, circumcision has been the fate of almost all American boys, and in spite of the diktat of the American Academy of Pediatrics that routine circumcision was unnecessary, the practice has continued. In Britain, circumcision has long been a prerogative of the wealthy. There are no problems in arranging for circumcision in Harley Street, but NHS surgeons are rightly reluctant and usually require medical rather than purely social reasons. In the 1970s, the British Medical Association came out positively against routine circumcision. Is it just conceivable that medical opinions on the matter might be ever so slightly influenced by financial considerations? Surgical circumcision is an easy and safe operation and can be properly done in about 15 minutes, either under local or general anaesthesia. A fashionable surgeon doing ten circumcisions in a day at $1,000 a time wouldn't be doing too badly. Nice work if you can get it.

The crime of Onan

It is doubtful whether anyone ever considered that masturbation could be medically harmful until a remarkable book was published in 1710. This book, written by a clergyman turned physician who chose to remain anonymous, was called Onania, or the Heinous Sin of Self-Pollution. It was an instant publishing success. In twenty years it had achieved no less than fifteen editions and by 1765 it had reached its eightieth. The book was more concerned with sin than with physical harm but, in those days, the two were closely interrelated and the book struck a resonant chord in the minds of its susceptible readership. From then on, masturbation was widely believed to result in all manner of diseases.

Influenced possibly by the success of this book, other books on the subject quickly appeared, the most notable being one by a Swiss physician, Dr Tissot, called *Onania, or a Treatise upon the Disorders Produced by Masturbation* (1758). Tissot's book was published in English translation in 1766, and, thereafter, there could be no doubt of the dangers of this vicious practice. Although neither of these books contained anything but straight assertion of pseudoscientific and pseudomedical dogma without a vestige of scientifically acceptable truth, nearly everyone, including the doctors, believed them.

Here is an unedited quotation from a family medical encyclopaedia, published in the 1880s: 'ONANISM – The crime of Onan – self-pollution – requires no further notice here, than to put parents on their guard respecting their children, in connection with this ruinous vice, acquired at school, and indulged in, in ignorance either of its sin or evil consequences. Some of the most lamentable instances of youthful decrepitude, nervous affections, amaurotic blindness, and mental debility and fatuity in early life, which come before medical men, are traceable to this wretched practice. Whenever young people, about the age of puberty, exhibit unaccountable symptoms of debility, particularly about the lower limbs, with listlessness and love of solitude, look dark under the eyes, &c., the possibility of vicious practices being at the root of the symptoms, should not entirely be lost sight of.'

Thousands of people suffered mentally as a result of the influence of pious statements of this kind. The Victorians were often frenzied in their anxiety over, and professed hatred of, the practice. During the early and mid-nineteenth century a spate of books on the subject appeared. Freud called it 'the primal addiction'. Many became seriously exercised over what they called 'spermatorrhoea'.

The French physician Lallemand described it as, 'A disease that degrades man, poisons the happiness of his best days, and ravages society.' The physician Spitzka wrote, 'There is a discrepancy between the results of natural and artificial excesses. Natural sexual excess has none of the perversions so characteristic of the latter. Nature has so arranged that there are limits to sexual excess. No such limits check the onanist.' In 1863, the Scottish physician David Skae was the first to identify what he called masturbational or masturbatory insanity.

One of the most vociferous against the practice was the English psychiatrist Henry Maudsley (1835–1918) after whom was named the psychiatric hospital in Denmark Hill, London. Maudsley published a paper on masturbation in the *Journal of*

Mental Science in 1868 in which he wrote of ' ... the high-pitched and absurd sentiments professed by these degraded beings...', and 'a mind enervated by vicious practices, dwelling continuously on sexual subjects. It is curious that to such a state of moral degradation have patients of this class come, that they will actually defend their vice on some pretence or other.'

The contemplation of female masturbation was too much for most of these gentlemen, and, for a time, the practice was deemed so heinous as to justify almost any remedy. Many women, detected in masturbation, were actually categorized as insane and locked up in mental hospitals. Others were forced to submit to mutilating surgery, especially removal of the clitoris (clitoridectomy). Doctors insisted that female masturbation was a cause not only of serious ill-health but also of insanity. Almost anything that could put a stop to it was justified. It is now hard to imagine the motives for such beliefs and attitudes, but the strength of them testifies to the power of sexuality in human affairs.

We can congratulate ourselves that we live in more enlightened times, in which most people understand that masturbation is no more harmful, and no less common, than sexual intercourse. The practice was almost certainly engaged in – no doubt guiltily – by most, if not all, of the men who devoted themselves so assiduously to its condemnation.

The Semmelweiss scandal

Ignaz Philipp Semmelweiss (1818–65) was the son of a prosperous Swabian German shopkeeper and was born in Buda, Hungary. He studied medicine at the Universities of Pest and

Vienna and in July 1846 was appointed as an assistant physician in the General Hospital in Vienna. At the time, nothing was known of the real cause of infectious disease. Germs were unheard of. Many doctors still believed in the assertions of Galen (see **Claudius Galen and the blood-letting disaster**) that infection was due to natural phenomena such as earthquakes, tidal waves, comets and eclipses of the moon. Others came nearer the truth and believed that they were due to the effects of decomposing organic matter.

There were two maternity wards in the General Hospital. In Ward 1, where the babies were delivered by medical students, the death rate from 'childbed fever' was horrifying – sometimes almost 30 per cent. In Ward 2, where deliveries were conducted by midwives, the rate was about 3 per cent. Childbed fever was a shocking condition in which young women, often in perfect health, developed a high temperature, severe abdominal pain, extensive red, inflamed patches in the skin (erysipelas), abscesses and collections of pus in the abdomen, chest and other parts of the body, severe prostration and then sank into a coma and death. Pregnant women begged and prayed not to be admitted to the notorious Ward 1. The doctors were well aware that cases of childbed fever tended to occur in clusters, but most of them considered that this was pure chance. Some of the more scholarly believed that such clustering was a natural phenomenon with a mathematical basis and cited the work of Daniel Bernoulli on the flatness of the solar system. Ironically, the American physician and author Oliver Wendell Holmes (1809–94) had produced clear mathematical proof that, if there was, in fact, no contagion, the probability against such clustering as was observed happening by pure chance was many millions to one. Holmes had thus concluded that there was some connection between the women who formed these clusters of cases.

Semmelweiss noticed that women admitted just after their baby had been born rarely suffered from the deadly disease. He was also deeply affected by the case of his friend and colleague Jakob Kolletschka, a professor of forensic medicine, who died after cutting his finger during a post-mortem examination. The changes found in Kolletschka's body were identical to those in the bodies of women who had died of childbed fever. Putting two and two together, Semmelweiss decided that the medical students must be carrying some poison from the corpses in the autopsy room to the labour ward. So he insisted that anyone delivering a baby must first wash his or her hands in chlorinated water. Within a year the mortality rate had dropped to one per cent.

Semmelweiss's chief, Dr Klein, and others, resented this interference and the suggestion that they might have been responsible for the women's deaths. Like other doctors of the time, they were proud of the 'hospital odour' they carried on their hands. In 1847 Semmelweiss outlined his ideas in a paper he read before the Vienna Medical Society. Little attention was paid to this. In 1850 Semmelweiss was forced out of his job, his work was forgotten, and the death-rate among the women rose again to record heights. Semmelweiss managed to get a job teaching midwifery at the University of Pest. While there, he conducted an extensive correspondence with leading European obstetricians.

In 1858 he wrote and published an article on the subject in a Hungarian journal. Finally, in 1861 he produced his great work – a book of 548 pages called *Die Aetiologie, der Begriff und die Prophylaxis des Kindbettfiebers* (*The Cause, Theory and*

Prevention of Childbed Fever). This remarkable book describes in detail all his work in Vienna and later in Pest. He also includes a great many of the letters he exchanged with other doctors. Unfortunately, this book is almost unreadable. It is badly arranged, repetitious, wordy and unclear. The arguments are weakeningly aggressive and reveal a distinctly paranoid attitude in the author. Ruthless work by a sensitive editor, able to sift the wheat from the chaff, would greatly have improved it and might have occasioned the saving of thousands of lives. Nevertheless, this book contains all the facts needed to demonstrate that Semmelweiss was right and had established that childbed fever was caused by contagion carried on the hands of doctors from one woman to another. It also contains unequivocal accounts of the transmission of infection from corpses in the post-mortem room to rabbits.

Here is a translation of a telling passage from this book: 'From the time of Hippocrates to the present doctors have believed that the fearful devastations which childbed fever has produced among women who have recently given birth, are to be ascribed to atmospheric influences. I was able, during the year 1847 in the great Vienna Lying-in Hospital, to show that this view was wrong, and that each single case of childbed fever was caused by infection. As a result of measures which I devised, I have had no epidemic in Vienna for 21 months, in St Rochus Hospital for six years and at the clinic in Pest for one year.'

Whether or not Semmelweiss was driven mad by the treatment he had received remains unclear. More probably, he had a psychotic tendency and was precipitated into a frank breakdown by professional disappointment and frustration. Be that as it may, he ended up in a mental hospital where he became violent and was beaten by the attendants. Two weeks later he died of blood poisoning from the injuries he had received. Fourteen years after his death, a notable French gynecologist was about to deliver a public lecture in Paris condemning the idea of contagion in childbed fever when he was interrupted and silenced by the great Louis Pasteur, who proceeded to announce his discovery of the organism responsible for childbed fever – the streptococcus bacterium.

Chloroform orgasms

In 1831, three scientists in three different countries – Samuel Guthrie in the United States, Justus von Liebig (of condenser fame) in Germany, and Eugene Soubeiran in France, almost simultaneously discovered and made an interesting new compound. Remarkably, each of these three chemists had, unknown to the others, mixed up some acetone with bleaching powder and added sulphuric acid. The result was a heavy, highly volatile, fragrant-smelling and sweet-tasting yellow liquid that proved to be an excellent cleaning agent for all kinds of stains. It could dissolve fats, oils, waxes and grease, rubber, gutta-percha and resins. It was called trichloromethane. Methane is a simple common gas consisting of an atom of carbon with four hydrogen atoms attached to it. If three of these hydrogen atoms are replaced by chlorine atoms, trichloromethane is formed. It is better known as chloroform. The liquid was easy and cheap to make and was sold as an effective spot remover.

In 1847 a Liverpool chemist called David Waldie, who had been experimenting with the effects of inhaling chloroform, decided that he would entertain his guests after a dinner party.

The results were spectacular and the party was a resounding, if somewhat soporific, success. The ease with which a person could be put to sleep by inhaling chloroform immediately suggested to Waldie that the drug could have medical uses. Soon afterwards Waldie met the celebrated Edinburgh doctor James Young Simpson. Simpson had been using ether to relieve the pains of childbirth but was dissatisfied with the results. The drug caused gagging and choking and had to be breathed for a long time before there was much effect.

Waldie immediately recommended chloroform and Simpson started to give it to his patients. The ladies were remarkably pleased but others were not. The next thing Simpson knew was that there was an outcry from the Church. Women, said the preachers, were meant to give birth in agony. This was clearly God's will – it said so in the Bible, 'And God said to Eve "In sorrow thou shalt bring forth children".' Even lay people – males presumably – were disgusted at the idea that women should be made unconscious at this important stage in their lives. This was clearly immoral. Feeling against chloroform ran high and, as may be expected, all kinds of stories were spread around. One of the most popular of these was that chloroform in moderate doses brought on erotic fantasies and converted birth into one long orgasm.

There was, however, one factor that quickly counteracted all these prejudices. On 7 April 1853 Queen Victoria decided that giving birth to her son, Prince Leopold, was getting to be altogether too agonizing and she asked for the celebrated Dr John Snow – the then leading expert on general anaesthesia – to give her chloroform. This was duly done and the Queen was so pleased that four years later she again asked for chloroform for the birth of Princess Beatrice. After this, all opposition to chloroform melted away. If the Queen approved of it, there was nothing more to be said. Dr Snow was lucky. Although unaware of it, he was running the risk of becoming one of the most notable medical blunderers of the century.

By about 1870, when chloroform was being extensively used as a general anaesthetic both for childbirth and for surgery, it was gradually becoming clear that this wonderfully pleasant and easy-to-take drug was not as safe as had been thought. A small proportion of patients who were given chloroform were dying suddenly for no apparent reason. Others were developing a disastrous liver condition known as acute yellow atrophy, from which most of them died. Later research showed that chloroform made the heart muscle exquisitely sensitive to the effects of adrenaline so that the beat became irregular and sometimes stopped.

Once it became known that chloroform was the cause of these tragedies, the drug fell into disuse and the doctors had to fall back on the much safer, if much less pleasant agent, ether.

Dr Battey and the epidemic of female mutilation

Robert Battey (1828–95), one of the pioneers of American surgery, got much of his early practice with the knife during the American Civil War. He was a surgeon in the Confederate Army and, during that exceedingly bloody conflict, operated on hundreds of gravely wounded men.

After the war Battey returned to his practice in Rome, Georgia, and turned his attention to women. He was a serious, scholarly man and soon built up a large and flourishing private gynaecological practice. In addition to becoming Professor of

Gynaecology at the medical college in Atlanta, Georgia, Battey set up a private hospital and, in his enthusiasm for his speciality, founded the Georgia Gynaecological Society.

What followed may seem to suggest that Battey became a callous, even bloodthirsty man, but this would be a mistaken judgement. Rather, the Battey story is a striking example of how incalculable harm can result from the highest motives and best intentions. Remember, however, that all this occurred in the 1870s when surgery was at a primitive stage, was highly dangerous, and had a high mortality from gross infection and internal bleeding. Most surgeons of the time considered that elective surgery – surgery performed other than for urgent life-saving purposes – was never justified.

One day Battey was asked by one of his medical colleagues to examine the latter's wife. This lady had, over the months, become, apparently, exceedingly fat. Closer inspection showed, however, that the increase in bulk was limited to the abdomen and that the lady, in fact, had an enormous ovarian cyst. Battey knew that these cysts, while by no means necessarily cancerous, could, nevertheless grow to a very large size and could prove fatal. After much discussion and consideration Battey decided to operate. On making the incision he was astonished at the enormous size of the tumour that pushed its way out of the wound. After quickly tying off its supplying blood vessels, Battey, with much-needed assistance, eased out of the incision a huge, fluid-filled cyst that tipped the scales at 30 pounds. The procedure necessarily involved the removal of the affected ovary.

By good fortune all went well, the woman survived and was, of course, delighted with her restoration to a normal shape and size. This success seemed to encourage Battey and he began to remove ovaries. Initially, he did this for obviously gynaecological conditions such as excessive menstrual bleeding. In those days, knowledge of the endocrine system was scanty. Thomas Henry Huxley's excellent book *Elementary Lessons in Physiology* of 1872, which contains a remarkably detailed and accurate account of all the other systems of the body, has nothing to say about endocrinology. So no one then really understood the effects of depriving young women of their oestrogen supply. In fact, no one knew that oestrogens existed. So if ovaries were removed, there was no question of hormone replacement therapy.

Battey's operation
In 1872 Battey was consulted by a strikingly beautiful young woman who was remarkable in that, although she had never had a menstrual period, she suffered every month from an episode of extreme abdominal pain and intense anxiety and mental distress. Battey decided that her body was trying to perform its natural menstrual function and that her monthly troubles could be relieved if her ovaries could be removed. It was well known that women without ovaries could not have menstrual periods. Battey's idea was entirely theoretical. The young woman also suffered from a serious inflammatory disease of the heart – endocarditis – and there really was no clear evidence of the cause of her monthly attacks. Before Battey could operate, however, the woman suffered a serious relapse and died. Post-mortem examination showed that she had been born without a womb.

This case had a profound effect on Battey who felt he had failed her. He was convinced that the attacks had led to excessive strain on her heart and was confirmed in his opinion that removal of her ovaries would have saved her life. He resolved that if ever such another case occurred, he would not hesitate. These were laudable motives for which he must be given credit. Before long, another young lady-patient appeared who seemed to qualify. This was a girl of twenty-three who, each time she had a period, developed convulsions and became almost comatose. In addition her periods were associated with painful hemorrhages in various parts of her body and she had developed a pelvic abscess. Her periodic pain was so severe that she had become addicted to morphine. With modern knowledge, it is easy to see that this girl was almost certainly suffering from the condition of endometriosis. This distressing disease features patches of womb-lining tissue in various places outside the womb – even in the brain – which, under the influence of the menstrual hormones, produce small local periods. Endometrial tissue is commonest on the ovaries and in the pelvis, but can occur anywhere.

It seemed obvious to Battey that this girl urgently required to have her ovaries removed. This was a reasonable and valid conclusion. Before operating, however, Battey discussed the case at length with the most distinguished gynaecologists of the time and the matter was debated at a meeting of the Boston Gynaecological Society. Finally, in August 1872 Battey operated and removed both ovaries. Not surprisingly, they were entirely normal. Battey went through a very worrying time in the days following the operation. He knew that if the woman died he might have to answer some embarrassing questions and might even face criminal prosecution. In the event he need not have worried. Although, as was almost inevitable in those days, the girl developed internal infection that proceeded to peritonitis – a common cause of death following abdominal surgery in those days – her immune system was able to throw this off and made a full recovery. The effect of the operation seemed miraculous. All her symptoms disappeared. She had no more fits, no more internal bleeding, and the abscess in the pelvis was absorbed.

Battey published an account of the case and this created a sensation in medical circles. Battey became famous and his procedure for the removal of the ovaries became widely known as Battey's operation. Gradually, Battey allowed himself to widen the indications for the procedure. Although he criticised many of his colleagues for doing this operation for unjustified reasons, the fact was that he, himself, came to consider that the operation was justified for a range of sexual disorders. Over the course of the succeeding years Battey gradually came to think that a wide range of conditions, including epilepsy, menstrual pain, nervous upset, nymphomania, and even insanity were due to ovarian dysfunction. The fact that most of the ovaries he removed were entirely normal did not deter him. He had the complete answer to this. Although the ovaries looked normal, he said, they could not be so as they were the cause of all these conditions. This masterpiece of circular reasoning is an excellent example of the way the reasoning function can be corrupted by power and success. Battey was the principal pundit of this new branch of medicine. He knew more about it than anyone else so he could not be wrong. Reason became replaced by simple assertion.

Many of Battey's colleagues were even less conservative than he was and took to the new ideas with enthusiasm. Oophorectomy – the medical term for removal of the ovaries – became the vogue procedure for all sorts of female complaints. New terms were coined. The diagnosis of *ovariomania* – any kind of psychotic or psychoneurotic disorder affecting women of child-bearing years – was commonly and solemnly applied to unfortunate young women and many of these had to submit to this mutilating operation. Many died and those who survived were sterile and menopausal, often in their twenties.

All this is on a par with the long-standing notion, originating with Plato, that many women's problems are connected with the womb. Plato believed the womb (Greek *hystera*) was a rather aggressive animal lodged in the woman's body and desperate to get on with its proper function of producing children. If, he taught, the uterus was long frustrated in this desire, it became angry and caused all sorts of upsets, especially emotional instability. Out of this rather quaint, male-oriented idea arose the later concept of hysteria – a condition in which bodily upset or loss of function arises without obvious organic cause. It seemed that, at least to the Deep South American doctors, hysterical disorders were somewhat old hat and that something new and more fashionable was called for – hence the concentration on the ovaries.

The idea that psychiatric disorders in women were caused by some disorder of the ovaries quickly caught on. Many psychiatrists, as anxious as anyone else to be in the forefront of medical advance, gave their approval to this view; some even insisted that all nervous and mental disorders in women originated in this way. This was all the surgeons needed. A positive epidemic of oophorectomy followed. This was justified not only on the grounds that it would cure these women but also because, as many of them claimed, sterilization would prevent the taint of madness from being passed on to the future offspring. Unfortunately, there was, at the time, a major vogue for eugenics. This had been started in England by Darwin's cousin

Francis Galton (1822–1911) and has been popularized by three books he published on the subject, in 1869, 1874 and 1892 (see **Eugenics in England**).

Spread of Battey's ideas

The Deep South of America was a fertile soil for the ideas that the race could be polluted by the influx of 'inferior breeds' and by the breeding of defective stock. So widespread removal of ovaries was an obvious step to improve the purity of the race. The idea quickly spread to the insane asylums. Here was obvious scope for surgery. In one asylum in Maryland, a special ward was set up for the women to have the operation. Oophorectomy was indicated, the doctors believed, for melancholy (depression), simple mania (often no more than attacks of hysterical behaviour), psychiatric upset following childbirth, epilepsy and other neurological disorders. Large numbers of women were operated upon. In a State asylum in Pennsylvania, fifty women were scheduled for operation when, fortunately, the Committee on Lunacy of the State Board of Public Charities got wind of it. These gentlemen had more sense than the surgeons and the psychiatrists and soon put a stop to this wholesale bloodshed. This did little to stem the tide of popularity for Battey's operation which was performed with undiminished enthusiasm on both sides of the Atlantic. It is difficult to know how many women were mutilated in this way, but in a paper published in 1906 in an American journal of obstetrics and diseases of women and children, it was estimated that about 150,000 had suffered this fate.

Gradually, towards the turn of the century, reasonable counsels began to prevail. Eminent British surgeons such as Spencer Wells (of artery forceps fame) and Frederick Treves (of Elephant Man fame) expressed scepticism and questions began to be asked. Regrettably, the idea that women's troubles were rooted in their wombs and ovaries was so firmly entrenched in medical thinking that it persisted well into the twentieth century. Some doctors seem to believe it to this day.

Removing the clitoris

One might expect, and hope, that, throughout history, doctors would be more free from prejudice against sexuality and its manifestations than lay people. One would be wrong. Doctors, for reasons best known to themselves, have often reacted with emotional savagery to the thought of female masturbation and, being possessed of the power to do so, have responded by making sure that this vicious practice is no longer possible. Masturbation (see **The crime of Onan**) was obviously a disease calling for the most stringent measures in its cure.

In the mid 19th century, the practice of clitoridectomy, a simple operation that any doctor could perform, was especially popular – with male doctors. At the time, the procedure was so well known that it even had a euphemistic term – extirpation. This vogue was closely related to the then current ideas that masturbation led to nymphomania, and nymphomania to the lunatic asylum. This was a wonderful piece of logical deduction based on nothing more than the observation that it was not uncommon to observe psychiatric patients in mental hospitals masturbating in public. Even some of the most eminent surgeons were, apparently, unaware of the logical fallacy in this. Unfortunately, these ideas, promoted by the medical Establishment were also widely accepted by lay people.

One of the most vigorous and enthusiastic promoters of clitoridectomy for masturbation was one Dr Isaac Baker Brown, a graduate of Guy's Hospital, a well known obstetrician and gynaecologist, a notable medical pundit and the author of one of the first textbooks on gynaecological surgery. In 1858 Dr Brown opened a private clinic in Notting Hill which was mainly devoted to the mutilation of women. In spite of the disapproval of his medical colleagues, Dr Brown advertised this clinic widely and effectively. It was so successful that the distinguished doctor resigned his official hospital appointment and moved over to full-time private practice. He became rich at the expense, in more than one sense, of many women.

Dr Brown was soon carried away by his enthusiasm for clitoridectomy that, in 1866, he published a handsome slim volume called *The Curability of Certain Forms of Insanity, Epilepsy, Catalepsy and Hysteria in Females*. This book contained accounts of 48 cases of female masturbation (Brown called it 'peripheral excitement') and the dire effects caused by it. This practice used up so much 'nervous energy' that it gave rise to a whole range of female disorders which he described with evident relish. All these conditions could be cured by clitoridectomy. The book is a farrago of imagined nonsense, misapplied observation and plain perversity of assertion based on prejudice. But Dr Baker Brown was high in the medical Establishment and, at least outside medical circles, his claims were believed. A report in *The Times* stated that Brown had 'brought insanity within the scope of surgical treatment'. The *Church Times* strongly advocated the book and recommended it to the clergy for the benefit of their flock.

The *British Medical Journal* had, however, by now had enough of the self-promoting Dr Brown. Even then, advertising was considered unethical and was frowned upon. A highly critical review appeared in the *BMJ* of 29th April, 1866. This review actually used the words 'female masturbation' and came down very heavily on the author for producing a work that had the appearance of books more commonly found on drawing room tables. Obviously Brown had intended that the book should have much wider than merely medical circulation and thereby promote even greater attendance at his clinic.

This review opened the floodgates for serious medical argument, much of which was critical of Brown. *The Lancet* joined in and was, on the whole, antagonistic. The attitude of the *BMJ* hardened into positive hostility against Brown and all his activities. *The Times*, ever ready to sway with opinion, now began to wonder whether it was legal for Brown to treat insanity. At that the Commissioners for Lunacy got into the act and began to investigate Brown's actions. In a panic, Brown denied what he had previously been claiming, and the *BMJ* reported gleefully that Dr Brown was now announcing that no patient of unsound mind had been cured of that disorder by clitoridectomy in his clinic.

Some big guns from the Royal College of Surgeons and the Council of the Obstetric Society now intervened, and Dr Baker Brown was told that he was liable to be expelled as a Fellow of the Society. Seriously worried, Brown declared that he would abandon the practice of clitoridectomy, 'pending professional enquiry into its validity as a scientific and justifiable operation.' The *BMJ* was, however, delighted to report that, in spite of this undertaking, Dr Baker Brown had continued to perform the operation. A meeting of the Obstetric Society was then held to consider Brown's position. Although he spoke eloquently, the whole tenor of the meeting ran against him and there were repeated accusations of quackery. When the vote was taken, 194 members voted for his removal and only 38 voted against his removal. Baker Brown was immediately expelled.

The extraordinary thing was that Baker Brown was disgraced, not because he practiced clitoridectomy for ridiculous indications, but because, out of greed, he had offended against professional ethics. No one ever suggested that there was anything wrong with clitoridectomy, as such. Many years were to pass before this operation was condemned by the medical profession.

Female circumcision today
The activities of misguided doctors, such as Isaac Baker Brown, are now, happily, a thing of the past, but it is important for people to understand that female circumcision is being practiced widely in many parts of the world, even in Britain, to this very day. Accounts of this barbaric practice appear in records dating back to before the time of Christ. Sir Richard Burton, who was never a man to conceal the truth, included an account of it in the manuscript of his book *First Footsteps in East Africa*, but his publisher, with characteristic timidity, cut it out. The term 'female circumcision' is actually a euphemism for genital mutilation, and is a cause of pain, humiliation and distress to millions of women living in male-dominated societies throughout the world. It is practiced in over 30 countries including sub-Saharan Africa, New Guinea, the Arab world, Australia, Malaysia, Southern Europe, South America, Western Asia and India. The prevalence rates in different countries range from 5 per cent to 99 per cent. Even women in Britain are not necessarily immune. Some 10,000 are currently at risk. It is estimated that at least 100 million women and girls alive

today have undergone genital mutilation.

Alleged motives for this abomination vary from place to place and various claims – religious, moral, even medical – are made for the social importance of the act. Women who have not been circumcised may be rejected as marriage partners. The real basis is probably the sense of male property in women that cannot tolerate the thought of female infidelity. Unfortunately, this motive is potentiated by the factor of cultural identity which, for many women, is of paramount importance. For this reason, women often submit willingly to the social pressures to accept circumcision – the alternative being ostracism. None of these reasons justify this cruel practice.

The procedure may involve removal of the clitoris only or may extend to radical removal of the labia minora and majora followed by stitching together of the raw surfaces so that they heal across and make sexual intercourse impossible. This major mutilation is called infibulation. It is done, usually between the ages of four and ten, but may be done at any age from one week to puberty. The usual procedure, in Africa, is for the girl to be held down on her back by a young man who lies under her, while two other people grip her ankles and force her legs apart. The operation is performed using a razor blade, a sharp ceremonial or other knife or a piece of broken glass. No attempt is made to sterilize these implements and no anaesthetic is used. Apart from the pain and suffering, female circumcision commonly leads to severe infection, bleeding, urinary infection, kidney failure from blockage to the outflow of urine, dangerous obstructed labor from tight obstruction to the vaginal outlet, tetanus and death.

The practice has been condemned by the World Health Organisation, the United Nations Human Rights Commission,

Unicef, the UN Children's Fund, the International Planned Parenthood Federation, the UN Convention on the Rights of the Child and other official bodies. It is illegal in Britain, Sweden, the Netherlands, and Belgium, but, at the time of writing, it is not yet illegal in the USA. A bill has, however, been presented to Congress. Despite this, and despite the efforts of many enlightened women who are campaigning against it, the practice goes on. In the west, such practices are rightly regarded as criminal assault, but it must be recognized that there are still many places where, in a context of male pride and a sense of property, the rights of women count for nothing.

A fatal shampoo

Dolores Behringer was seventy-two and still very attractive. She was also more than usually conscious of her appearance and spent a great deal of time and money on beauty care. She was especially proud of her hair, which was remarkably thick. There was little natural tint in it these days, but her weekly shampoo and colour rinse attended to that. She would have been hard pressed to say what colour her hair was.

Recently, however, her shampoo sessions had been less enjoyable than usual and she had almost come to dread the moment when she was asked to bend her head far back over the washbowl. Gradually she had come to realize that, in this position, any turning movement of her head was liable to cause trouble. Sometimes she just felt a little dizzy, sometimes quite severely nauseated. On one occasion, she had found that one side of her face was quite numb for several hours after the hairwash. She had never suffered any permanent ill effects and simply put the problem down to advancing age. The experience was, however, becoming so unpleasant that she decided, reluctantly, to speak to the girl about it.

On her next visit she found to her surprise that her usual girl was absent and that a stranger was in her place. Feeling rather shy, she decided to say nothing. The new girl was a little rough and was rather inclined to push her about, but Dolores was never one to complain. While her hair was being rinsed, the girl twisted her head sharply to one side to keep the soap out of her eyes. Dolores suddenly realized that she did not know where she was, that she could not speak properly or find the right words and that she was profoundly dizzy.

She struggled to get up and promptly fell out of her chair. The new girl called her a stupid old bitch and tried to help her to get up, but Dolores was paralysed. At once the whole salon was in a panic and a doctor was called. By the time he arrived Dolores was feeling a little better and was able to give some kind of an account of her symptoms. But before the ambulance came she had a second and more severe attack and in spite of all the paramedics could do, she was dead on arrival in hospital.

After investigation and autopsy, Dolores' death was attributed to a severe reduction in bloodflow along the vertebral arteries of the neck. This was the result of the position adopted for shampooing her hair. The vertebral arteries help to supply the brain with blood, and, like other arteries are nearly always affected, in elderly people, by the common arterial condition of atherosclerosis. The 'beauty parlour stroke syndrome' has been reported in neurological and in general medical journals, but is not widely familiar. Doctors who have investigated it recommend that the practice of extending the neck in beauty parlours should be abandoned and should be replaced by the much safer flexed posture.

Marie Stopes and the contraception debate

Marie Stopes was born on 15 October 1880, in Edinburgh, of intelligent, middle-class parents who had met at a meeting of the British Association for the Advancement of Science. Her father, Henry Stopes, was an engineer and architect whose real interest – whipped up by the then revolutionary theories of Darwin, Lyall and Thomas Henry Huxley – was archaeology. Some of his archaeological discoveries, however, ran so strongly against the account of the creation of the world in the book of Genesis in the Bible that clerical objection forced him to withdraw a paper he had prepared for the British Association. Henry was an attractive, charming and sexy man. But he had the misfortune to marry a woman eleven years older than himself to whom sex was a disgusting and painful duty to which she was expected, unwillingly, to submit but could not be expected to enjoy. Any accidental sexual gratification was to be considered a matter for shame. Charlotte was a hard, cold woman who, after visiting her husband on his deathbed, wrote to him: 'The sensual look has passed away from your face that so pained me, and you seem to have regained the chastened expression of your youth.' Notwithstanding a most unhappy sex life, the couple did succeed in having children, and Marie was the first.

Marie Stopes was an exceptionally bright young woman who was educated at schools in Edinburgh and London and, in 1902, took a First Class Honours degree in botany at University College, London. While there she became President of the Women's Debating Society and shocked the University authorities by instituting joint debates with the men. Two years later, after working with a Professor Goebel in the Botany

Department of Munich University, she took a Ph.D., and in 1905 took a D.Sc. diploma in London. Marie was the youngest Doctor of Science ever to qualify in Britain. Both in Germany and in England she quickly acquired a formidable reputation for hard work and was thought attractive by her colleagues. She was slim but full-breasted with a mass of dark, reddish-brown hair and large, down-sloping, hazel-coloured eyes. Unorthodox – some said shameless – in her dress, she favoured floating, Pre-Raphaelite drapes that emphasized her femininity and revealed her figure. She was also strongly passionate.

She had little time for the German men however, with their machismo and assumptions of male superiority, but while working in Professor Goebel's laboratory she met a thirty-seven-year-old Japanese researcher called Kenjiro Fuji. They fell in love and, when she returned to England, Fuji followed her. This attachment survived a spell when she was a lecturer at Manchester University and a separation of eighteen months after Fuji's return to Japan. They had planned to marry in 1907 and in July Marie sailed for Yokohama. She then suffered a kind of Madam Butterfly in reverse. Fuji's feelings seemed to have changed; he alleged that he was unwell and finally contrived, allegedly, to develop leprosy so that he could, without loss of face, be released from a liaison he no longer wished. Sadly, after a year and a half in Japan, Marie returned to England.

In 1911 Marie met the Canadian geneticist Reginald Ruggles Gates at a scientific congress in St Louis. He was two years younger than her and of a reserved and sensitive character that immediately attracted her. She was also greatly attracted by his scientific attainments in the then new field of genetics, and was not indifferent to the fact that he had a private income. A week after they met, Gates proposed and she accepted him. In spite of the passionate and poetical wooing of Professor Fuji, she was still a virgin. Marie did not change her name and insisted that she should still be called Dr Marie C. Stopes.

The marriage was a disaster. Gates was impotent and Marie knew nothing about sex, so was unable to help. Conflict between the demands of their respective careers – Marie was not going to settle down as an obedient housewife – and Gates' violent, jealous rages and envy of her professional superiority, soon raised strong tensions. Marie desperately wanted a baby but actually did not know how to go about it and was unaware of the reason why she did not become pregnant.

Then the distinguished writer and translator of Tolstoy, Aylmer Maude, who was estranged from his Russian-born wife fell for Marie and moved in with them. For a year they continued as an extraordinary *ménage a trois* while the handsome and charismatic Maude, twenty-two years her senior, systematically but platonically demonstrated to her, by his wooing and his explanations, the inadequacies of her marriage. Eventually, Gates threw Maude out of the house but by then the marriage was over in all but name. Marie actually wrote a play about the whole situation which was considered so scandalous that the Lord Chancellor refused it a performing licence. Thomas Hardy found the plot incredible.

Sexual research

At this point Marie decided that it was high time she learned something about sex. So she went to the British Museum Reading Room and ploughed through everything she could find on the subject in three languages. She also worked her way through textbooks on the physiology of human reproduc-

tion. Astonishingly, as a Doctor of Science and a world authority on palaeobotany she knew practically nothing about this
until she undertook these studies. Most of the sex books in the
BM library were in the 'restricted access' section but Marie
insisted on seeing them and, because of her professional status,
was allowed. The most influential of all this reading were the
works of Havelock Ellis: *Man and Woman* (1894) and *Studies
in the Psychology of Sex* which was completed in 1910.

Marie was still a virgin in October 1914 and was thus in a
position to file a petition for nullity of marriage, rather than
divorce, on the grounds of non-consummation. This petition
was not heard until two years later and although the costs had
gone against her husband, he had left the country and Marie
paid them. She was very hard up at this time, as her salary as a
lecturer at University College was barely enough for her to live
on. In the meantime, however, her private studies into sex were
bearing fruit. She had for years been possessed of strong literary ambitions and, apart from her many professional papers,
was constantly engaged in creative writing. She wrote a good
deal of poetry, eight or nine plays, a musical comedy and a film
script. None of these were quite what the public wanted and
none were performed. Now, carried away with the importance
of what she had been reading in the BM library, acutely aware
of how much it meant to her, and very conscious of the repressive climate of the times on all matters sexual, she was fired
with the impulse to pass on to others some of this new and
exciting knowledge. The result was the book *Married Love*.

For the times, this book was alarmingly frank. It contained
frightening words like 'orgasm', 'ejaculation', and 'intumes-
cence' and advocated mutual masturbation in pregnancy. Most
remarkable of all, it actually indicated that women, like men,

experienced sexual desire. Not surprisingly, a number of publishers were thoroughly frightened off. One or two were disgusted, and said so. The realist Sir Stanley Unwin saw the commercial potential of the book and wanted to publish it, but his colleague C.A. Reynolds disagreed. All these people presumably regretted their timidity. When the book was finally published by the small firm of A.C. Fifield in March 1918, it sold over a million copies.

Married Love is not exactly a scientific book and it contains a good deal of imaginative nonsense. Marie was not above making up what she thought ought to be true. Also, since she was still a virgin at the time she wrote it, there was a quality of poetical romanticism about the book that real experience would probably have dispelled. None of these criticisms is of the least importance in relation to the impact this book made on the lay public. It was a book that was desperately needed, and for the first time the facts of life were laid plain for the ordinary man and woman.

Wealth and fame

At the age of thirty-seven Marie was married for the second time to Humphrey Vernon Roe, brother of A.V. Roe who founded the Avro aviation company. Alliot V. Roe was a successful inventor but ran into serious debt with his early ventures into flying. Humphrey agreed to settle his debts in exchange for a half share in the Avro company. His timing was immaculate. This was 1914. Avro, of course, became immensely important during the First World War and by 1918 had produced 10,000 aircraft. By then, both brothers were comfortably off. It was at that point that Humphrey met Marie Stopes.

Marie's book made her famous with the majority of the public and infamous with a prudish and prejudiced minority. The correspondence she received from the public was enormous and immediately made apparent to her how strong was the general desire for sexual knowledge. This was not prurience – although for many, no doubt, there was an element of that – but a genuine and proper anxiety to know, and, perhaps, to dispel the mountain of guilt that had been heaped up by the Church around the subject. This correspondence also made it plain that there was a huge desire for knowledge on contraception. For large numbers of women, mainly but not exclusively those in the poorer classes, annual pregnancies were a nightmare that were destroying their lives and their health. Constant childbearing was also, for many, a serious economic problem. Marie was not long in doing something about this damaging situation. At the end of 1918 she published *Wise Parenthood*, a guide to family planning. This book had, however, actually been written before *Married Love* was published and was not, as she disingenuously claimed, a sequel unwillingly written in response to public demand.

The fact that she made this claim reveals her nervousness about the book. She had good reason. In this book, not only did she advocate and explain contraception, she also had the temerity to suggest that sex was a good thing in its own right and that regular sex had a human function quite apart from the question of the production of children. This book, too, was far from scientific. Although Marie did not think much of the 'safe period' method of contraception, she, like the whole of the medical profession, was so ignorant of the physiology of sex that she thought it was midway between two menstrual periods. This was unfortunate, as this is actually the time when ovulation occurs and pregnancy is *most* likely to result. She was also mistaken in suggesting that a cervical cap might safely be left in place for long periods. Marie favoured the tight cervical cap over the larger diaphragm, then widely known as the 'Dutch cap'. She was convinced that the diaphragm would stretch the vagina and prevent the woman from exerting vaginal grip on the penis, during sexual intercourse, which she considered most important. There is no basis in this belief.

Church, press and professional reaction
Wise Parenthood brought the issue of contraception right out into the public domain and brought down a storm of protest and criticism on the head of the audacious and reckless author. Even the *News of the World* was outraged and offered a free willow-pattern tea tray as a congratulatory gift to all mothers of ten children. Not to be outdone, the *Daily Express* ran a prize competition for Britain's largest family. The editor of *New Witness* expressed his feelings in scurrilous terms: 'The peculiar horror of her book is that it is couched in pseudo-scientific terms, and is addressed to the married woman.' The novelist Arnold Bennett had written a foreword to the fifth edition of the book. This particularly angered the *New Witness* editor: 'Mr Arnold Bennett [should] at once dissociate himself from Dr Marie Stopes and her rubber goods. The introduction he has written to her filthy book is a disgrace to him and to his (and our) profession.' The magazine *Plain English* wrote: 'Evidence has reached us which goes to prove that Stopes has, by means of her disgusting books, done an inconceivable amount of injury.'

The Roman Catholic Church was, of course, strongly antagonistic to any work that promoted contraception and Marie was attacked from many quarters. One apologist actually insisted that passing on syphilis to the baby was less of a sin than using contraceptives. Another described her writing as 'a most profane compound of imaginary mysticism and pornography', and stated that he would pray to God 'to prevent your doing the amount of harm to others – in body and soul – which your expedients are calculated to produce.'

The reaction of the medical profession was, on the whole, no less critical. While Marie certainly had support from some doctors, many were passionately against her. Possibly the fact that she was not medically qualified may have influenced some, but it was mainly on moral and dogmatic grounds that she was opposed by the doctors. Some of their attitudes were extraordinary. Dr Amand Routh, the consultant obstetrician at Charing Cross Hospital insisted, with no grounds in medical fact, that artificial methods of contraception caused pelvic problems, nervous exhaustion and inability to concentrate. Other doctors claimed that they caused neurasthenia, menstrual disorders and even neuralgia. Women who used contraception were liable to become 'prurient, foul-mouthed and foul-minded with advancing years.' Another doctor threatened to ask his MP to try to promote legislation for the suppression of such 'rubbish'. The distinguished physiologist, Professor Sir Leonard Hill, FRS., one of the principal medical pundits of the time, claimed that women who used contraceptives lost their looks early and became thin and neurotic.

First clinic

Although Marie was deeply conditioned by her middle-class values and was capable of a remarkably patronizing attitude to the 'lower classes', she was profoundly affected by the evidence provided by the voluminous correspondence and controversy aroused by her books. This evidence soon convinced her that millions of women, mainly of the working class, were suffering terrible hardship, ill-health, loss of the quality of life and premature ageing as a result of the physical and psychological burdens of continual child-bearing. This was an issue that became, for her, of central concern and the more opposition was aroused by her views, the more determined she became to promote them and to see them implemented. So, in 1919, with the support of her husband, she decided to set up a birth control clinic. This was called The Mothers' Clinic for Constructive Birth Control.

The clinic was not an immediate success. In the first nine months, only a little over 500 women had attended. There were considerable objections to it from the doctors. Their ignorance can be summed up in a comment in *The Lancet* of 26 March 1921 to the effect that qualified doctors might inform themselves of the relative degree of nervous wreckage to be anticipated from the use of any one method of contraception. *The Lancet* is probably the most prestigious medical journal in the world and would claim to reflect current medical knowledge and opinion. Dr Anne McIlroy, Professor of Obstetrics and Gynaecology at the Royal Free Hospital chaired a meeting of the Medico-Legal Society at which she gave a paper attacking contraception. In her summing-up she instanced, as an example of the joys that contraception would deny, the happiness of the large Irish peasant families.

Action for libel
One of Marie's most vociferous critics was a Dr Halliday G. Sutherland, a Scot who had been converted to Roman

Catholicism. In a book condemning birth control he described Marie as a 'doctor of German philosophy' who had opened a birth control clinic in London at which working women were instructed in a method of contraception described by Professor McIlroy as 'the most harmful method of which I have had experience.' He went on to express his amazement that 'this monstrous campaign of birth control' should be tolerated by the Home Secretary. 'Charles Bradlaugh,' he added, 'was condemned to jail for a less serious crime.' Sutherland also accused Marie, in effect, of treating poor women as subjects on which to experiment. Marie brought an action for libel.

The trial opened in the High Court on 21 February 1923 before Lord Chief Justice Hewart. Marie was called and spent three hours in the witness box under intense examination by defence counsel. Although the attack on her motives and beliefs was almost continuous and was intended to ridicule and discredit her, she bore up wonderfully well. She was an excellent and quick-witted public speaker and gave as good as she got. Unfortunately, the other witnesses on her side were not always so effective, and some of them did considerable harm to her case. As the trial proceeded it became increasingly apparent that the judge, although quicker in his grasp of the matter of the case and clearer in his exposition than some of the counsel, was, in fact, a monster of prejudice. In addition, the defence was obviously more effective than counsel on Marie's side. Her own counsel, Mr Patrick Hastings, started out with a brilliant opening speech and then seemed to lose interest. Indeed, towards the end of the nine-day trial, Marie was openly quarrelling with him and was having to insist that he ask her certain questions.

The jury came to a very confusing conclusion. They found

that the words Marie had complained of were defamatory, but that they were true. They did not think that they were fair comment and awarded damages of £100. This was generally supposed to indicate a victory for Marie Stopes but the judge deferred his decision until the next day. Most of the papers assumed that Marie had won but the judge decided otherwise and gave his decision in favour of Dr Sutherland. It then appeared that the jury had intended to find in favour of Marie. Nearly all the newspapers deplored the judge's decision.

This trial brought Marie so much sympathy and general approval and the effect of the publicity on the sales of her books was so great that it soon became apparent that she had done far better by 'losing' than she would have done had she won. Even so, she appealed against the judgement and five months later Justice Hewart's judgement was reversed. Marie was awarded the £100 damages, half the costs of the actions and the whole cost of her appeal. These financial matters were important to her. Marie had been running the whole costs of her clinic out of her own pocket and was by no means as wealthy as most people supposed.

But the Catholic Church, which was supporting Sutherland and meeting his costs was not finished yet. The defence appealed to the House of Lords and the Catholics brought all their big guns to bear on the case. A fund was set up 'to give the country a lesson of the solid Catholic determination to stem the flood of Pagan ideas which threatens the future of the Nation and of Christianity. Every Catholic – every right-thinking person – is asked to give something – something large if possible.' With a remarkable show of ecumenicism, the Anglican *Church Times* invited its readers to contribute.

The judgement again went against Marie, and the costs, of

about £12,000 were awarded against her. She even had to pay back the £100 she had been awarded in the first appeal. The anti-contraceptionists, both clerical and medical, were jubilant. To their fury, however, the remarkable publicity generated by the trial and the appeals, and the great public sympathy for Marie, worked strongly to her advantage. Her book sales increased substantially, attendance at her clinic rose to a record figure, in the year of the trial, of 2368, and public opinion began to swing in favour of contraception. When, soon afterwards, she wrote the soberly professional and restrained book *Contraception, its Theory, History and Practice* expressly for the medical and legal professions, the doctors, with few exceptions welcomed it and it was well reviewed in the medical press.

The trial and the appeals also greatly increased her correspondence, mainly from women appealing for help and from those who wanted to thank her for what she was doing for them. One postal delivery alone amounted to 350 letters. The battle against prejudice was by no means over, but the corner had been turned.

The DES disaster

DES is diethylstilboestrol, a synthetic female sex hormone that was first produced in 1938 and promoted in the late 1940s. DES appeared under various trade names such as Estrobene, Cyren A, Domestrol, Stilboestroform, Sexocretin, Sebol, Biodes, and so on. There were at least 28 different trade names for the same preparation. DES was manufactured by many companies and was widely used for many years. It was given by mouth, by intravenous injection, and by vaginal pessaries and creams. It was even included in cosmetics and skin creams sold over the counter.

DES was prescribed for a variety of conditions including oestrogen deficiency, unwanted lactation and a tendency to spontaneous abortion. Ironically, DES is now known to have no useful effect in preventing abortion but it was in the hope of so doing that the drug was given to so many women in early pregnancy. DES was also extensively used in veterinary medicine and in livestock farming for the caponization of chickens and to increase weight gain in young cattle, sheep and pigs. It was even used as a contraceptive in dogs.

In 1971 a paper appeared in the *New England Journal of Medicine* showing the association between maternal treatment with stilboestrol and cancer of the vagina in the daughters of women who had, much earlier, taken the drug. Intensive research followed and it was discovered that not only was DES useless in preventing abortion but that exposure of the foetus at an early stage to this and other synthetic oestrogens could, if it survived and grew up, have a number of serious effects on it after puberty, especially in females. These included adverse changes in personality and behaviour; depression and anxiety; menstrual irregularity and infertility; probably excessive pituitary gland secretion of the milk-promoting hormone prolactin; and, worst of all, abnormalities in the womb, cervix and upper vagina including vaginal and cervical cancer.

Forty out of 60 women who had been exposed to the drug were found to have a T-shaped womb. These distressing complications occurred in the daughters of women who took DES while they were pregnant. Most of the women who developed cancer were 20 to 25 at the time it was detected, but some were younger. The incidence was somewhere between 1 in 1,000 and 1 in 10,000. It was also found that DES could produce genital abnormalities, but not cancer, in male offspring of women who took the drug. Ironically, DES is still used to help to treat certain cancers of the breast and cancers of the prostate gland in men.

Prohibition
In the United States the drug was prohibited for use in pregnancy in 1971. In Britain it was not until 1973 that the *Committee on Safety of Medicines* advised that it should not be used in pregnancy. By then an estimated two to three million American women had received the drug during pregnancy, and a survey in Britain indicated that about 7500 women had taken it, mainly during the 1950s. The women themselves suffered no significant ill effects but had to wait, sometimes for as long as 30 years, before discovering whether their children were affected. By then, of course, most of those who had had the drug were unable to find out which drug manufacturing firm had supplied it. This made it very difficult to bring legal claims for damages, but courts in the USA, sympathetic to the plight of these women, introduced various ways of circumventing this impediment to justice. In America, some women even tried to bring legal actions as the granddaughters of women who had taken DES, but such actions were deemed inadmissible by the New York Court of Appeals.

Soon legal actions began to succeed. In the case of one woman who made a successful claim against the American drug manufacturer Eli Lilly, the jury awarded $2 million to her and a large sum to her husband. The judge, however, proposed that she should have $200,000 a year for the next 51 years – a total of over $10 million. It seemed almost certain that the drug firm would appeal against this award and the case would have dragged on. So, on 17 October 1991 the woman settled for $4,250,000. This was by far the largest sum paid out for a DES damages claim.

In Holland, where many thousands of affected women had banded together in a society called *DES Action* to bring claims against eight drug firms, the courts initially insisted on strict proof and these mass claims failed. In 1992, however, the Supreme Court ruled that it was unfair that compensation should be denied because a drug company had ceased to exist or that appellants could not name the company concerned. Following this decision lawyers hoped that every affected woman would receive £37,000. The drug firms were horrified and pointed out that claims of this size would be ruinous and would, at best, seriously interfere with innovative research.

The DES story, like the thalidomide tragedy, underlines the dangers of taking drugs in pregnancy, especially when the body organs are at an early stage of development and the tissues are most sensitive to damage.

Sex change

Tammy Beadle was undoubtedly a man. A test had shown that every cell in his body contained an X chromosome and a Y chromosome. So he had to be a man. Or had he? Unfortunately, Tammy's genitalia had been ambiguous at birth and he had been reared in a gender opposite to that of his true biological gender. When this happens, the gender in which the child is reared is nearly always the one he or she accepts and wishes to retain. This is what had happened to Tammy. Tammy's parents had assumed that he was a girl and had, at first, raised him as a girl. All the experts will now tell you that the gender assumed by parents and by the individual during the critical early period of life will nearly always become definitive in the mind of the person concerned.

It was not until everything started to change at puberty that the truth about Tammy became painfully apparent. Tammy's equipment soon grew to respectable dimensions and it became all too apparent that he was, anatomically, an unequivocal male. So his embarrassed parents started putting him in boy's clothes. This was especially disconcerting and humiliating for Tammy's father, who was a doctor. It was worse for Tammy who hated it and knew that it was all wrong. He grew up in a real mess, psychologically and, although his academic performance had been excellent and he ended up with a good degree in electronics, his social problems made it very difficult for him to settle to a career. His father refused to listen to any talk on the subject and was unsympathetic to what he thought were Tammy's unreasonable objections.

Tammy finally got a job, however, maintaining the computers in a large London business organization. This was well below his level of potential but he earned enough to be able to leave home and live his own life, which he did with marked relief. He was sorry to leave his mother who had responded kindly to his distress, but felt little regret at leaving his father. Soon after he moved he began to dress as a woman during the evenings and weekends. This caused quite a lot of trouble, especially with his landlord, who called him a 'fucking pervert'. Unfortunately, someone from the office saw him and the news got around. His boss had him in and warned him that any more trouble of that kind and he was out.

Transsexuals and gender identity

As a result of his parents' mistake, Tammy was a transsexual. Transsexuals are people who are anatomically normal but who feel that they belong to the sex opposite to that of their bodies. This has nothing to do with homosexuality or transvestism, although, naturally, transsexuals often wish to wear the clothes of the opposite anatomical sex. The conviction that they are of the wrong sex is often so strong that they feel they are in an alien body. Most of them are willing to go to any lengths to change it, and Tammy was no exception. His own GP was sceptical and about as unsympathetic as his father. He tried to send him away with the advice to 'pull himself together'. But Tammy was persistent and eventually got as far as a sex counselling clinic. From there, he was referred to a hospital unit specializing in sex change surgery.

At the gender identity unit he was advised that sex, or gender, was a complex entity that could not simply be established by checking whether the chromosomes were of the female (XX) configuration or the male (XY) pattern. Knowing that he was genetically male, Tammy agreed fervently with this. He was also told that no surgeon would contemplate sex change surgery until completely satisfied that the person concerned was genuinely transsexual. This, too, met with Tammy's unequivocal approval, for he was quite clear in his mind that he was transsexual.

The surgeon he was seeing was impressed by his history and his attitude and was willing to take the matter further. So Tammy then had a long and careful investigation by an experienced psychiatrist. Her report showed that Tammy was entirely free of any psychiatric disorder and that any psychological trouble he had had was the result solely of the disparity between his anatomical sex and his mental outlook. Tammy was persistently uncomfortable about the inappropriateness of his anatomy and had, for several years, been preoccupied with the desire to get rid of his appurtenances. He was also deeply desirous of acquiring breasts. At the conclusion of her study, the psychiatrist said to Tammy, 'It's not often that I say this, but in your case, I really think you should come over to my side. I don't think you will regret it. That's what I'm going to recommend.'

Tammy was deeply moved and, with tears in his eyes, gave her a long, grateful hug. The psychiatrist remained smilingly unperturbed by this unprofessional encounter.

Surgery

Her report was considered by the surgeon and deemed sufficient justification to plan for surgery. But before this was done Tammy was given a course of female sex hormones and a drug that countered the effects of his own male hormones. He was delighted with the result of this treatment. The texture of his skin became finer, his breasts enlarged nicely and the contours of his hips became wider and more rounded. A breast implant operation was then done and, from that time on, Tammy took permanently to women's clothes and began to refer to himself as a woman. This meant that he had to give up his job, and, for a time, was out of work. But living on the dole and moving to cheaper lodgings seemed unimportant in comparison with the amazing sense of greater normality he/she now felt.

Tammy had a few more interviews with the surgeon who seemed to be reluctant to go further, but in the end he/she was scheduled for operation. With an immense sense of easement, Tammy was finally relieved of those parts that now seemed to her, more than ever, a hideous and ridiculous disfigurement. In the course of the operation the surgeon also fashioned for her a pair of labia and an artificial vagina, just in front of which was the new opening for the urethra. It was some time before she got accustomed to sitting down to have a pee.

As soon as she had recovered from the operation Tammy started to look for a new job. Her somewhat masculine appearance and her inexplicable reticence about her past history were against her and it was some time before she was taken on. But when she did start to work, no one was in any doubt as to her competence, energy, reliability and value. The firm was concerned with the development and production of CD-ROM disk drives for personal computers and within a year she had moved from the technical to the managerial side.

In her second year, she took a three-week holiday during which, at her own expense, she had plastic surgery on her nose and ears. When she returned, she was immediately aware of the new sexual currents running in the office. This amused and pleased her but she had never been much interested in sex and had little trouble coping with harassment. The feeling of most of the men towards her remains one of considerable respect tinged with attraction and an intriguing sense of challenge over her apparent indifference. She has recently been the subject of a head-hunting bid by another firm and seems set for a highly successful career as a business executive.

Her only major setback was when she visited her parents, now in their fifties, to bring them up to date with developments. Tammy's father was furious. Having gone through the emotional and professional trauma of having a girl turn into a boy, it was altogether too much for him to have to cope with the boy turning back into a girl again. Her mother just looked at her, gasped and then embraced her warmly. Daddy was unable to conceal his emotion: 'You have disgraced me, and you have disgraced your mother. You are an unnatural, disgusting ... person. Good God! I don't even know whether to call you a man or a ... How can I ever mention to any of my colleagues that my ... my son ... is now ... I wish you had never been born.'

Hysterical blunders

The idea of hysteria has always been popular with men and goes back a long way. Plato taught that the womb (Greek hystera) was a rather aggressive animal lodged in the woman's body and desperate to get on with its proper function of producing children. If it was long frustrated in this desire, it became angry and caused all sorts of upsets, especially emotional instability. Out of this rather quaint, male-oriented idea arose the later concept of hysteria – a condition in which bodily upset or loss of function arises without obvious organic cause.

The popular idea of hysteria – a dramatic emotional outburst, with loud crying and perhaps inappropriate laughter, and a fairly obvious attempt to attract attention – is not exactly what doctors mean by the term. Today, we define hysteria as an upset of body function not caused by an organic medical condition, but resulting from purely psychological disturbance or need. The affected person is, to all appearances, unaware of the psychological origin of the problem. Because the term is recognized as having elements of political incorrectness about it, kindly doctors have sought a new name for it. The current euphemism is 'conversion disorder'. There is also, for the same reason, a growing tendency, especially in America to refer to hysteria as Briquet's syndrome. As in the case of all euphemisms, however, it is only a matter of time before these terms, too, are thought of as being just as objectionable as the term hysteria. So there is really not much point in changing the terminology.

The condition is much more common in women than in men and is more likely to affect people of poor educational, occupational, economic and intellectual status than the more fortunate. It usually appears in the late teens and rarely starts after the age of thirty. Research has failed to produce any convincing evidence that hysteria is hereditary. The condition does not, apparently, run in families, and if one of a pair of twins has hysteria, the other is very unlikely to show any such tendency. Male relatives of hysterical women have been shown to have somewhat increased rates of antisocial personality, alcoholism and drug abuse. Most British psychiatrists agree that hysteria is not hereditary.

Origins

The most obvious example of the origin of hysteria is the conflict between sexual or aggressive impulse and social prohibitions. At a time – as when Freud was formulating his ideas – when such prohibitions were much stronger than they are today, hysteria was commonplace, and people like Freud were greatly impressed and influenced by it. Today, because sex – or at least discussion of it – is out in the open, hysteria is comparatively rare, and represents only about one psychiatric case in ten thousand.

Conversion is said to provide a means of disguising the

impulse from the person concerned, so that it need not be confronted, and, at the same time, communicating to others, without actually saying anything, that there is a need for special attention. Unacceptable life situations may be changed, other people may be conveniently manipulated, responsibilities may be evaded. These effects are called secondary gains.

Common physical effects are loss of sensation, paralysis, tics and jerks, blindness, deafness and epileptic-like fits. Significantly, hysterical neurological disorders usually correspond to no possible anatomical pattern – there is, for instance, no nerve disorder that could possibly cause loss of sensation affecting only the glove area of the hands. People with hysterical blindness do not bump into things and those having hysterical fits do not hurt themselves when they fall. In spite of claiming to be grossly disabled, people with hysteria often show remarkable unconcern. This is known as *la belle indifférence* and is a feature of the condition.

Mass hysteria

Mass hysteria is a strange phenomenon that has been surprisingly common throughout history. It is an eloquent testimony to the power of suggestion and to the ease with which hysteria can affect the most apparently normal. Most cases seem to be based on a common conviction which influences behaviour. As in other forms of hysteria, women are affected more often than men. A crowd of young girls at a celebrity pop concert will readily become convinced that the men on the stage possess all the most wonderful and desirable qualities – something that, to the detached observer, is manifestly not the case. There can be no questioning the sincerity of the emotions felt by these fans. A crowd of worshippers at a religious meeting will begin to suffer convulsions after one person is affected in this way. Girl's schools have quite often had fainting epidemics. Many women in Mattoon, Illinois, reported having been anaesthetized and assaulted by an unknown prowler when suffering from mass hysteria.

Examples

One of the most impressive, and well-documented cases occurred in a clothing factory employing many women workers. After a consignment of foreign cloth arrived, some of the women began to complain of insect bites that caused such severe general upset that they had to stay off work for a few days. Enquiries by researchers showed that those who were affected had been working very long hours of overtime to get enough money to meet their family obligations but were conscious of their neglect of their families. Some solution had to be found to the dilemma. The most searching investigation failed to show that any insects were present, but the factory had to be closed and fumigated.

The Salem witch trials in Massachusetts in 1692 revealed one of the most notorious examples of mass hysteria, in which increasing numbers of people became convinced that they were being bewitched after two young girls began to behave strangely. Nineteen people were hanged and one pressed to death with stones.

For various reasons it is easy to feel antagonistic to people we suspect of hysteria. Hysteria implies dishonesty, attempts at manipulation and a seeming desire to achieve an advantage without earning it. We are also apt to disapprove of people whose behaviour is emotional, dramatic and exaggerated. Reactions of this kind can readily cloud our judgement. It is only after considerable experience with the person that one can come to a reliable and fair decision about hysteria. Such a decision should not be followed by automatic condemnation and rejection. People who produce hysterical symptoms have real problems that may be harder to solve than those caused by organic disease. However threatening they may seem to our equanimity, and however negatively we may tend to view them, they deserve our sympathy. Some doctors frequently describe patients as hysterical; others try to avoid the term. Some even hold that its use is simply an indication of a derogatory attitude to certain patients – nearly always women – and indicates male chauvinism.

For all these reasons, hysteria has been, and continues to be, the occasion for a great many medical blunders. It is very dangerous for a doctor to assume hysteria and to fail to carry out a full neurological examination. Genuine neurological disease is now much commoner than psychologically induced disorder, and the signs of organic disease are sometimes so improbable as to suggest hysteria. Numerous cases have been reported in which a perhaps hasty diagnosis of hysteria has led to delay in making the correct diagnosis and providing timely treatment for an organic disorder. Such a mistake can sometimes lead to serious consequences for the patient, and is unpardonable.

Once a clear diagnosis of hysteria is established, the affected person can safely be treated by a careful exploration of the origins of the problem. In most cases the symptoms clear abruptly after a fairly short time, but often the underlying cause remains. Further conversions, taking either the same or different forms, are common, especially in those who have much to gain.

Vicarious menstruation

The word 'vicarious' is normally used to refer to something done or experienced on behalf of another person. A royal whipping boy, for instance, suffered punishment when the prince was naughty. Vicarious menstruation in this sense, however, would be somewhat mind-boggling. The term has been in use for at least 100 years and the condition it describes – menstrual bleeding from a site other than the vagina – has been recognized for about 2000 years.

The first-century Roman physician Aulus Cornelius Celsus, whose book *De Medicina* was one of the first medical texts to be printed, wrote: 'Women in whom the blood fails to submit to menstrual discharge will often spit it out. According to the medical authorities, blood may come from ulceration of any part, or from its rupture or from the opening of the termination of any vein.'

Frederick Hoffmann
One of the earliest detailed reports of this condition was that of the Swiss pathologist Frederick Hoffmann (1610–1742). In a book about abnormal bleeding, Hoffmann wrote: 'A 30-year-old woman, at the time of menstruation, was overtaken by a grave sensation of anxiety. At that, the flow of blood stopped and a sense of heaviness in the chest and palpitation of the heart ensued. At the time of the next menses, only a small trickle of blood appeared, *per via naturalis*, but this was accompanied by a feeling of heaviness and oppression in the chest and pain in the back and under the lower ribs. For four days she coughed up blood. Thereafter, whenever she menstruated, she brought up blood from the lungs. This varies in quan-

tity for five or six days. This continued for nine years. Whenever menstruation stopped by reason of pregnancy, the coughing of blood also ceased, but returned soon after childbirth, in its accustomed turn, even during lactation. This woman's health remained good, but it was in vain that she did seek advice and cure, from the doctors, of this bleeding from the lungs.'

Hoffmann was hard put to explain this phenomenon but made a valiant effort. He concluded, he said, that there must be a 'regurgitation of blood from the womb to the chest.' This, he thought, was the result of the anxiety, occasioned by the menstrual period, widening and laying open the lung blood vessels and thus allowing the blood to escape. With termination of the menstrual period, there was no excess blood in the chest and the vessels were able to close. With repetition, nature formed a kind of habit and the effect occurred more easily.

Reports of vicarious menstruation indicate that the lungs are by no means the only alternative route for the discharge of blood. Various ancient writers have cited cases in which blood emerged from all the other orifices of the body and from some other places. There are reports of vicarious menstruation from the nose, ears, eyes, stomach, breasts, finger, umbilicus, bladder and rectum. In the light of modern knowledge, some of these sound more plausible than others. There is also a strong general tendency to fail to refer to the fact that, in most of these cases, bleeding must also have been accompanied by a normal menstrual period. We now know that this must have been so, but it seems that many of the early writers were convinced that the vicarious site of egress ought to be an alternative to the vagina. In accordance with the common principle of bending the facts to accord with the cherished theory, at least some of them would underplay the normal menstrual flow that accompanied the more interesting phenomenon. Also, a study of many of these reports indicates that they were, in fact, simply cases of abnormal bleeding from various sites in women who happened, for various reasons, not to be menstruating. In addition, unfortunately, a study of early medical writings shows that these scholars were as much given to plagiarism as are modern writers and the number of different cases of genuine vicarious menstruation described is much less than at first appears.

There seems to have been a general opinion among ancient physicians that vicarious menstruation was, on the whole, a good thing. Most of them held that menstrual blood was dangerous and had to be discharged somehow if the health of the woman was to be preserved. So if it could not get out through the natural channel, it was desirable that it should get out some other way. The male idea that menstrual blood is 'unclean' has, of course, been widely held since the mists of antiquity and this was reflected, perhaps unconsciously, in earlier medical opinion.

So, wherein lies the blunder? All the evidence to explain the strange phenomenon of vicarious menstruation was available to any ancient doctor interested enough to perform a post-mortem examination on a woman with the condition. In fairness, it must be said that, although the condition that gives rise to menstrual bleeding from abnormal sites is quite common and is well recognized today, it is not at all common for the bleeding to occur externally.

Here are the facts:

Endometriosis

Endometriosis is an extraordinary condition involving the presence, in abnormal sites, of the tissue that is normally present only as the lining of the womb. This tissue is called endometrium. In this disorder, endometrium may occur in the fallopian tubes, on the ovaries, deep within the muscular wall of the womb itself, scattered about the interior of the pelvis, or even in such remote sites as anywhere in the abdominal or chest cavities, in the lining of the nose or in the lungs.

Wherever it may be situated, endometrial tissue is affected by the hormones that control the menstrual cycle. It therefore goes through the same sequence of changes that affects the womb lining, including the monthly casting-off of blood, mucus and surface tissue. Because the blood and other material produced at these abnormal sites cannot usually escape, there is a local build-up of pressure, and pain occurs with each menstrual period. Accumulation is especially likely with ovarian endometriosis and there is a tendency for large ovarian cysts to develop. These can attain a considerable size and sometimes persuade the affected woman that she is pregnant. When such ovarian cysts are removed they are found to be full of a dark chocolate-coloured fluid. Up to half of all infertile women have endometriosis.

The symptoms of endometriosis are, of course, abolished by pregnancy and by the menopause. This suggests a method of treatment and they can readily be controlled by the continuous use of oral contraceptives or by any other measure that suppresses the function of the ovaries. A complete cure, however, will usually require surgical removal of the patches of endometrial tissue wherever they might be.

Chapter Three

Fighting plagues

The plague and the dogma

Plagues have ravaged mankind from the dawn of history. Thucydides (471–400 BC) in his *History of the Peloponnesian War* provides a graphic description of an epidemic – probably pneumonic plague – in Athens in 430 BC. 'No healing art,' he records, 'was of any use, nor were prayers, consultations of the oracles or anything else. Men in perfect health were seized in a moment with violent fever, inflammation of the eyes, sore throat and tongue. The breath was foetid, there was coughing and vomiting, violent convulsions, livid skin breaking out in pustules and ulcers. The internal fever was intense so that the sufferers could not bear to wear even the finest linen garments, but insisted on going naked. They longed for cold water; many threw themselves into the cisterns. There was an intolerable restlessness which never left them. Either they died on the seventh or ninth day or, if they lived, the disease descended into their bowels where it produced violent ulceration, severe diarrhoea, and later exhaustion that carried them off. The fury with which it fastened on each sufferer was too much for human nature to endure.'

The Black Death – the popular title for bubonic, pneumonic

or septicaemic plague – is a disease of rats that is spread to man by rat fleas discouraged by the death and cooling of their hosts. There were epidemics in Rome in the years AD 68, 79, 125 and 164. The latter epidemic lasted for 16 years and threatened to destroy the army. Tacitus records that 'the houses were filled with corpses and the streets with funerals'. Another devastating outbreak occurred in south-eastern Europe in 6 AD. Up to one third of the population of the Byzantine Empire may have died.

Famous plagues and estimates of death
The Black Death – mainly bubonic plague – appeared again in Europe in 1347. After such an interval it found a highly susceptible population. For four years the plague took a greater toll of life than any previously recorded disaster. Spread to Europe it is said to have been caused deliberately by Chinese or Mongolian (Kipchak) soldiers, besieging a trading post in the Crimea, who catapulted plague-infected corpses into the town. The disease appeared the same year in Sicily and the following year in North Africa, Italy, Spain, France and England. A year later it was appearing all over Europe and soon spread to Scandinavia and the Baltic states, ravaging populations wherever it arose. Further outbreaks occurred at intervals over the succeeding fifty years, the last in 1400.

The virulence of the disease varied. Estimates based on local archives suggest that between one-eighth and two-thirds of the affected populations died from it. The contemporary French historian Jean Froissart (1333-1419) believed that about one third of the population of Europe – some 25 million people – succumbed. This estimate is generally accepted. The population of England halved during the period of the plagues. Local depopulation was ubiquitous: a thousand villages disappeared. There were too few labourers to cultivate the land and much farmland was abandoned. Landowners were ruined. Wages and prices were forced up. Serfdom had to be abandoned. In spite of panic measures introduced by the Government to freeze wages, the surviving peasantry enjoyed greatly improved conditions.

Regrettably, the doctors were of very little help. To most of them, as to the churchmen, the visitation of the Black Death was seen as God's punishment for sin. This view was reinforced by religious teaching and men were taught to accept the horrors with resignation and to await the end of the world, which the plague presaged. Many accepted this teaching and tried to deflect divine wrath by prayer, fasting and self-flagellation. Many gave all their possessions to the Church. Not all were so amenable. Faced with the imminent threat of death many decided to get what pleasure they could out of life and adopted a philosophy of *carpe diem*, 'Let us eat, drink and be merry for tomorrow we die.'

Inevitably, the Jews, who were hated for their usury and were blamed for most things, were accused of being the cause of the plague or of being responsible for spreading it. They were claimed, on absurd evidence, to be poisoning wells or practicing black magic. Pogroms, torture and execution abounded and thousands were burnt in supposed retaliation. Many who owed them money were content to pass by without protest.

In 1348 Pope Clement VI granted absolution from all sin to any who should die on a journey to Rome where, in defiance of the plague, a Holy Year was being celebrated. By Easter, well over a million people from all over Europe had gathered in

Rome bringing with them an enormous sum of money in offerings to the Church. They also brought the plague with them. Inevitably, the disease spread through the crowds. A million people died. The Pope, on excellent medical advice, had sequestered himself in a room in Avignon, and survived.

The plague of 1664

In 1664 the plague returned to England. Again, any immunological resistance had been lost by the passage of time. Daniel Defoe records in his *Journal of the Plague Year* how in December of that year '... two men, said to be Frenchmen, died of the plague in Long Acre, or rather the upper end of Drury Lane ... in the last week in December 1664 another man died in the same house, and of the same distemper.' Over the ensuing weeks a steady rise in the number of deaths in the city alarmed the inhabitants. Pepys records in his diary: 'June 7th – The hottest day that ever I felt in my life. This day, much against my will, I did in Drury Lane see two or three houses marked with a red cross upon the doors, and "Lord, have mercy upon us," writ there.' By mid-July the weekly mortality bill showed 71 deaths from the plague in Tower Hamlets, but this was nothing to what was to come. In the week 8 to 15 August 3,880 deaths from the plague were recorded. The figures for ensuing weeks were: 4,237, 6,102, 6,988, 6,544, peaking in the week September 12th to 19th at 7165. Between 8 August and 10 October 49,705 people died of the plague.

Again Pepys: 'December 31st – Many of such as I knew very well, are dead; yet to our great joy the town fills again, and shops begin to open again. Pray God continue the Plague's decrease ... '

Pepys' prayer was answered and the numbers of deaths fell

as rapidly as they had risen. Nine months later London suffered the worst fire in its history, but a great purification. Between 2 and 5 September 1666, much of the city, including 13,000 houses, was destroyed.

It is extraordinary to recount that, in spite of the evidence before their eyes, hardly any of the medical men of the time seemed to consider that the plague could be infectious or contagious in the sense we now understand the terms. There was one exception to this blundering lack of common sense, and the writings of this man were available to them from the middle of the sixteenth century. Girolamo Fracastoro (1478–1553) was a Veronese poet, mathematician, physician, astronomer, geographer and pioneer of epidemiology. He is best remembered for his poem about the shepherd Syphilis, called *Syphilis or the French Disease*, which tells of the misfortunes of a young man smitten with the disease by Apollo. This was the origin of the medical term. Fracastoro had, however, a much more important claim to fame. In his book *De Contagione et Contagionis Morbis (On Contagion and Contagious Diseases)* which he published in 1546, he showed clearly that diseases such as the plague could be transmitted from person to person by mere association of bodies or of clothes.

Fracastoro went further and concluded that there must be very small bodies or 'germs' – he called them 'seminaria' – which carried the disease from person to person. This was an idea of the first importance and its application could have saved millions of lives. Unfortunately, the doctors were too influenced by dogma, both medical and religious, to pay any attention to Fracastoro's well-reasoned arguments. It must be accounted as one of the greatest medical blunders in history that they ignored the opinions of this brilliant man.

Dr John Snow and the Broad Street pump handle

Here is an excellent instance of a serious medical blunder arising because of unthinking acceptance of medical dogma in
spite of it being contrary to reason. Medicine, like other professions, has been, and still is, at the mercy of authoritarian pundits whose views have to be accepted because of the status of
the person who asserts them.

Cholera is a highly infectious disease caused by an organism
known as the *Vibrio cholerae*. Nowadays, we think of cholera
as a tropical disease but there was a time when this disease was
common in Britain. Symptoms start one to three days after
infection and the first sign is the abrupt onset of painless, but
profuse, watery diarrhoea and vomiting. Soon there is severe
dehydration from fluid loss. The cholera organism produces a
toxin which damages the whole lining of the small intestine,
causing inflammation so intense that some of the mucous
membrane inner lining of the bowel flakes off. This produces
the characteristic 'rice-water' stools by which the disease is
often recognised. There is severe thirst, weakness, wrinkling of
the skin, intense, cramping muscle pain, and, in about half of
the untreated cases, death.

Treatment of cholera
Cholera occurs in epidemics in areas of poor sanitation,
because it is spread by contaminated water supplies or food
contaminated by the excreta of people with the disease. It can
easily be avoided if nothing is taken which has not been boiled.
Moreover, the condition is self-limiting and recovery occurs in
three to six days if the amount of fluid in the body can be kept
reasonably high.

Water and salt replacement is the essential element in the treatment and if this is effectively done, survival and full recovery should be assured. It is not always possible, however, to replace fluid sufficiently by mouth, and intravenous infusion may be necessary. Antibiotics, such as tetracycline, are effective against the organisms, but are no substitute for efficient fluid replacement. Cholera vaccine is effective, but regular booster injections are necessary.

The remarkable Dr John Snow (1813-58) was a Yorkshireman whose medical career began in Newcastle-upon-Tyne when he was apprenticed, in 1831, to a local surgeon. He was soon very busy, for Newcastle was in the grip of a devastating cholera epidemic. Snow had to watch helplessly as hundreds of his patients died of the terrible outpouring of watery diarrhoea which left them so depleted of fluid that they could not maintain their blood circulation. The experience left a deep impression on Snow and when he moved to London he made a special study of cholera, at the Hunterian Medical School, in the hope of discovering how it was spread. At the time, almost all doctors believed that cholera, like malaria, was spread by 'bad' air. Snow, a man of original and thoughtful mind, decided that the uncritical acceptance of this theory was illogical. Something in the air might affect the lungs, but why should it cause a disease that primarily affected the intestinal tract? Snow decided that the spread of the disease was much more likely to be the result of something swallowed.

Snow's studies of 1849
In 1849 a major cholera epidemic occurred in London. With his new theory in mind, Snow decided to investigate, and he did this to some purpose. In his paper *On the Mode of*

Communication of Cholera, published that year, he wrote: 'The most terrible outbreak of cholera which ever occurred in this kingdom, is probably that which took place in Broad Street, Golden Square, and the adjoining streets, a few weeks ago. Within two hundred and fifty yards of the spot where Cambridge Street joins Broad Street, there were upwards of five hundred fatal attacks of cholera in ten days.'

Snow went on to relate how he suspected the 'much-frequented' street pump in Broad Street, and, when he inspected the water from it, found small, white, flocculent (fleecy) impurities floating in it. These, although he did not then know it, were, in fact, shreds of cast-off intestinal lining from cholera patients that had been passed in their stools. Snow then conducted a detailed analysis of the deaths and showed that only people who drank from this well contracted cholera. Those using other nearby wells did not. Later it was shown that the brick lining wall of a sewage cesspool only three feet from the Broad Street well was cracked and leaking, allowing the contents to get into the water in the Broad Street well. Snow recommended that the pump handle be removed. This was done and new cases immediately stopped occurring.

In 1854, Snow proved that cholera could be caused by faecally-contaminated water from the river Thames. It was not, however, until years later that his contribution to epidemiology and preventive medicine was fully appreciated.

Snow later became a pioneer in the use of general anaesthetics and achieved a major breakthrough in acceptance of the method when he administered chloroform to Queen Victoria in two of her labours. After the publication of his book *On Chloroform and Other Anaesthetics* in 1858, pain relief in childbirth became respectable (see **Chloroform orgasms**).

Their Lordships' delays

James Lind was born in 1716, the son of a prosperous, middle-class Edinburgh family. At fifteen he was apprenticed to an Edinburgh physician and at twenty-three he joined the Navy as a surgeon's mate. The same year the war between England and Spain began and Lind saw much service on board ship.

What he saw there appalled him. Although the officers enjoyed tolerable conditions, the seamen lived in dreadful squalor. Their quarters were cramped, perpetually wet, mouldy and rat-infested. The stink, compounded of dry rot, dead rats, putrid food and filthy men, was unbelievable. Fourteen inches of sleeping space was allowed each man in which to sling a hammock. There was no question of washing either the person or the clothes and both were invariably lousy. Clothes soon became ragged. The seamen's diet consisted exclusively of measly salt pork and beef, ship's biscuits and foul drinking water.

Scurvy

Although many of the officers seemed indifferent to these conditions, Lind was not. As a student of hygiene, he was not in the least surprised that there was so much sickness on board, in particular the dreaded scurvy from which the death rate was horrifying. This disease fascinated Lind. The officers appeared to be largely immune, but the men suffered terribly. First the gums would become crumbly and would bleed on a touch, then great purple bruises would appear spontaneously in the skin. The arms and legs would swell up and the joints would become abominably painful so that the least movement was a torture. In the later stages of the disease, the breath became foul, the teeth came loose and fell out, and one's strength failed so that standing became impossible. Those who reached this stage usually died, often from pneumonia.

Lind soon discovered that no one had the least idea of the cause of scurvy. He also discovered that the disease was a far more important cause of human suffering and bereavement than warfare, shipwreck, accident or drowning. It was killing more seamen than all these other causes put together. Between the years 1500 and 1800 more than a million seamen died from scurvy. Ashore, the disease was rare. Theories as to the cause of scurvy abounded. Every naval surgeon had his own ideas and was convinced that he was right. But these ideas were so variable and contradictory that none could be believed. Lind decided to find out.

Lind's experiments

Just about the only thing he knew about the causation of the disease was that, in general, it only affected people on long sea voyages who did not go ashore for many weeks at a stretch. Lind thought about this and about the fact that scurvy was rare ashore and concluded that it must have something to do with diet. In May 1747, convinced that this was the cause, he instituted a series of tests. A full report of these tests can be read in his journal. He selected twelve men suffering from scurvy to an approximately equal degree of severity and put them all together in the forehold. They were all given the same basic diet, but to this was added six different supplements. Each day, two men were given a quart of cider; two were given vinegar three times a day; two had twenty-five drops of *elixir vitriol* three times a day; two were given half a pint of sea water; two were given cream of tartar purgation together with a medicine recommended by a hospital surgeon consisting of garlic, mustard, balsam of Peru and gum myrrh; and two were given two oranges and one lemon every day.

Results

At the end of six days, one of the sailors who had had the fruit was actually fit for duty, the other was greatly recovered and was fit enough to become the nurse to the rest. The test was continued for two weeks but none of the other men showed any improvement. Lind was convinced. There was something in the fruit that was capable of curing scurvy. Anxious to spread the news, he retired from the Navy and went to study for a doctorate in medicine at Edinburgh University and to write a book on the subject of scurvy. In 1750 he became a Fellow of the Royal College of Physicians and in 1753 his classic work *A Treatise on the Scurvy* was published in Edinburgh. Three further editions of this book came out in the succeeding twenty years.

Delays

It was one thing to write a convincing book, but quite another to convince their Lordships of the Admiralty. Although Lind was appointed Chief Physician to the new Royal Naval Hospital at Haslar, Portsmouth, and published another major work entitled An Essay on the Most Effectual Means of Preserving the Health of Seamen in the Royal Navy, his work was ignored by the only people in a position to put it into universal practice. Fresh fruit was expensive, there were logistical problems, the proofs were not particularly convincing. So, while Lind continued for twenty-five years to work at Haslar, treating more cases of scurvy and making many other contributions to medicine, their Lordships – eating like princes in the

London clubs – did nothing and thousands of seamen continued to die each year.

Dr James Lind died in 1794 and never saw the results of his work put into practice. Perhaps he could have been more forceful in Whitehall. Maybe he should have banged a few tables – or a few heads. His pupils, Blane and Trotter, to whom he had unequivocally demonstrated the effectiveness of his method, were, however, more insistent, and succeeded. In the year following Lind's death an order was issued by the Admiralty that every British naval seaman should have a spoonful of lime or lemon juice each day. From the time that this order was implemented scurvy disappeared from the Navy. So it was nearly fifty years after Lind's discovery of the means of preventing and curing scurvy before anything positive was done.

The British 'limeys' had other things to thank Lind for. During his time at Haslar, he managed to persuade the Admiralty that regular washing and clean uniforms were a good idea; he showed how safe drinking water could be obtained from sea water by distillation; and he arranged for medical examination of recruits and introduced the use of cinchona bark (which contains quinine) against malaria.

The active ingredient in fruit and vegetables that prevents scurvy is, of course, vitamin C, but this was not isolated until well into the twentieth century. The American biochemist Charles Glen King achieved this feat in 1932. The vitamin had been recognized for some time and its relationship to scurvy was acknowledged in the name ascorbic acid, given to it by the English chemist Sir Walter Norman Haworth when, two years later, he succeeded in synthesizing it. We now know that ascorbic acid is essential in the proper maturation of the body's main structural protein, collagen. If one's diet is deficient in vitamin

C, weak collagen is formed with the result that blood vessels and other tissues readily give way. The collagen strands that hold teeth in place soften, and bleeding occurs into the skin, muscles, and joints.

Very little vitamin C is needed to promote healthy collagen and this quantity is readily obtained from any normal well-balanced diet. Nowadays the limeys are so well fed that no supplement is needed.

Linus Pauling and the vitamin C blunder

Linus Pauling (1901–94), twice a Nobel prize-winner, was one of the most distinguished scientists of the century. His book *The Nature of the Chemical Bond and the Structure of Molecules and Crystals* revolutionized chemistry and has been described as one of the most influential science texts ever written. He played a major part in laying the foundations of modern chemistry, biochemistry and molecular biology. He adapted chemistry to quantum mechanics and pioneered several fundamental methods of determining molecular structure. *New Scientist* described him as one of the twenty greatest scientists of all time, on a par with Newton, Darwin and Einstein. Most people would agree that Pauling is no fool.

Pauling's theories on Vitamin C
In 1970 Pauling published a little book called *Vitamin C and the Common Cold* in which he expressed the opinion, based on careful observation of his own experience, that regular fairly large daily dosage of this vitamin, i.e. amounts well in excess of the minimum required to prevent deficiency, would produce

'an increased feeling of wellbeing, and especially a striking decrease in the number of colds caught, and in their severity.' Pauling examined previous trials of the method, most of which had produced disappointing results, and pointed out that the dosage that had been given in these trials was nowhere near large enough. In spite of his persuasive arguments Pauling was dismissed by many of his colleagues, and by most of the medical profession, as a crank. Very few if any doctors believed that there was anything in the vitamin C story and there were plenty of pitying smiles whenever Pauling's theory was mentioned.

Professional scepticism

So far as the doctors were concerned, the idea had been adequately tested in a number of well-conducted trials and no useful effect had been shown to occur. No one seemed to pay any attention to Pauling's point about the importance of the dosage of vitamin C. Everyone knew that Pauling had a large jar of ascorbic acid powder on his desk and regularly crunched away at it. There were raised eyebrows at the reports that he was eating several grams of the stuff each day. Everyone knew that you needed only about 20 mg to prevent scurvy. Linus Pauling was being ridiculous. Such a pity that so brilliant a man should sink to such nonsense ...

That is how matters stood for ten years or so, and then the unexpected happened. In the late 1980s something new and very important began quietly to emerge in medicine. This was nothing less than an understanding of the way human cells, tissues and organs were damaged, not only in minor disorders like the common cold, but also in major conditions like heart disease and cancer, and even in ageing. The literature on this subject in the medical journals grew steadily, but around 1992 it suddenly erupted. Many hundreds of papers were published, and continue to be published in increasing numbers in journals like *The Lancet*, the *British Medical Journal*, the *New England Journal of Medicine* and the *Journal of the American Medical Association*. The interest was so great that at least one completely new journal, devoted exclusively to the subject, was produced. The general scientific journals like *Nature and Science*, the specialized biochemical and molecular biology journals, and the popular science magazines like *New Scientist* and *Scientific American* have also published widely.

Free radicals
All these original papers and reviews indicate that this vital tissue damage is caused by microscopic groups of chemicals, known as free radicals, which are naturally produced in enormous numbers in the body. Free radicals also occur in cigarette smoke, car exhaust and industrial fumes and are generated in the body when it is exposed to ultraviolet light from the sun and to other forms of radiation. Produced in excess and not checked, the destructive effect of free radicals on body cells and thus on many tissues and organs can be very serious. Their role in the causation of the arterial disease atherosclerosis, that leads to most cases of heart disease and other serious conditions such as gangrene, is now well understood. Atherosclerosis, incidentally, is the number one killer in the Western World, and claims more victims than any other single cause. The damaging effect of free radicals on the heart muscle after a heart attack is also clear. An enormous amount of research has shown that free radical damage is implicated in a wide range of other diseases and disorders. These include:
- Coronary thrombosis

- Angina pectoris
- Heart failure
- Stroke
- Brain damage
- Ageing
- Kidney disease
- Cancer
- Inflammatory disorders
- Cataract
- Poisoning
- Radiation sickness
- Rheumatoid arthritis
- Male infertility
- Retinopathy of prematurity
- Malnutrition

This alone is a major medical advance that has already begun to have an important impact on the understanding of disease processes. But this is not all. There is now strong and increasing evidence that the damaging effects of excess free radicals can be limited or even prevented by taking large doses of antioxidant substances such as vitamin C and vitamin E. Beta-carotene, the antioxidant provitamin A has also been shown to be an important weapon against free radicals. Beta-carotene is the stuff that makes carrots orange and is converted by the liver into vitamin A.

Free radicals do their damage by a common chemical process known as oxidation. Today, no one questions that antioxidant substances can 'mop up' free radicals and prevent them from damaging cells. Vitamin C is one of the best known and most effective biological antioxidants. Already, the subject of free radicals is getting to be big news outside scientific circles. Essential facts that the scientists have known for several years are gradually coming together to form a picture that may well transform medicine, and these facts are beginning to filter through to non-scientists. More and more references to the subject are appearing in newspapers and magazines.

So it really begins to look as if Linus Pauling might have been right after all. What a pity he did not live long enough to have the satisfaction of knowing that, at last, the doctors are having to admit that it was they, not he, who had blundered.

Typhoid Mary

A carrier is a person who breeds the organisms of an infectious disease in his or her body, and passes these on to infect others while remaining immune to the disease. The most notorious carrier of all time was 'Typhoid Mary'.

Mary Mallon, of Oyster Bay, Long Island, contracted typhoid some time around the turn of the century and made a full recovery. In 1901 she got a job as a cook to a family in New York City. A visitor to the house and the family washerwoman contracted typhoid. In 1902 Mary moved to another family job. Two weeks later two other servants developed typhoid, then all seven members of the family. In 1904 sporadic cases of typhoid began to occur in Oyster Bay and adjacent towns and these soon developed into an epidemic. Investigation showed that the sources of the infection had one thing in common – they all came from households in which Mary Mallon had been cook. Fifty-one direct cases were proved to have arisen in this way, three of which died.

Countless other secondary cases occurred.

In 1906 Mary took service with another family and six members succumbed to typhoid. At this point suspicion fell on Mary, but when she was confronted with this uncomfortable fact, she promptly disappeared. In 1907 she turned up as cook in a house in Park Avenue, Manhattan, but again fled before she could be apprehended. At length she was caught and was put into hospital under supervision. She promised never to work again as a cook and to report for regular checks. Both promises were soon broken, however, and she was committed to an isolation centre on North Brother Island, off the Bronx. In retrospect, it was thought highly likely that she had been the primary source of the Ithica, New York, typhoid epidemic of 1903 in which there were 1,300 victims.

Mary was a tough-minded woman who knew her rights. She appealed to the United States Supreme Court but was retained on the island until 1910 when she was released on condition that she would never again take employment as a food handler. This, as it proved, was a real medical blunder.

In 1914, epidemics of typhoid broke out among the staff of a New Jersey Sanatorium and a Manhattan Maternity Hospital. Mary had worked as a cook in both and had left in a hurry without giving a forwarding address. She was finally traced to a private house in Westchester County where she was living under an assumed name. In the interests of public safety, Mary was committed to be detained in North Brother Island where she died in 1938.

Typhoid carriers are people who develop a permanent infection in the gall bladder where the *Salmonella typhi* organisms breed freely without causing any apparent harm to the host. These bacteria pass down the bile duct with the bile and enter the intestine where they contaminate the bowel contents and are excreted with the faeces. Thus the stools of typhoid carriers are heavily infected with typhoid organisms. So, in the course of normal activity, are the fingers. If such people do not wash their hands scrupulously after visiting the toilet, these unwelcome and invisible agents are inevitably passed on to others. Unfortunately, food handlers are not always noted for the high standards of their personal hygiene, and, as in the case of Mary Mallon, unwanted donations are to be expected from time to time.

The hemophiliac HIV disaster

Hemophilia is a condition causing a life-long tendency to excessive bleeding with very slow clotting of the blood. The term is a somewhat ironic reference to 'loving blood'. Hemophilia is due to the absence of Factor VIII, one of the many elements necessary for normal blood coagulation. It is a recessive genetic disorder, the gene being on the X (sex) chromosome. The sons of a hemophilic man do not suffer the disease and do not pass it on to their descendants. All the daughters carry the gene on one X chromosome but, because the gene is recessive, do not suffer the disease. They are, however, carriers, and there is a 50 per cent chance that the X they transmit to their sons will be the one with the hemophilic gene. So, on average, half their sons will suffer from hemophilia. Female hemophiliacs are very rare and occur only if hemophiliacs marry carrier females.

In hemophilia, bleeding occurs either spontaneously or on

minor trauma, most commonly into the joints, causing severe pain, swelling and spasm of the associated muscles. The blood absorbs within a few days and the symptoms settle. Repeated episodes, however, lead to damage and chronic joint disability. Bleeding may also occur into the bowel, causing symptoms which mimic other acute abdominal emergencies and problems from excessive blood loss. External bleeding, from injury, whether accidental or surgical, continues indefinitely unless special measures are taken to stop it. Dental extraction is followed by very prolonged bleeding. The severity of hemophilia varies with the level of Factor VIII activity in the individual and in severe cases this may be less than 2 per cent of normal.

All of these troubles can be prevented by giving one or other of two special factors, called Factor VIII and Factor IX to keep the condition in check. Unfortunately, these factors are active only for a short period so repeated injections are necessary. Hemophiliacs are advised to try to avoid trauma, but to lead as normal lives as possible. The anti-hemophilia factors are derived from donated blood and are present in such low concentration that several thousand donations are necessary for the preparation of a single batch. Factor IX has always been available in sufficient quantity in Britain, but Factor VIII is scarcer. In 1973, the scarcity was such that the British authorities decided to import Factor VIII concentrates from America. These were made from the blood of paid donors. So each hemophiliac person who injected himself or herself with this material was exposed to blood products and possible contamination from the blood of some thousands of other people.

By the end of June 1985, five hemophiliacs in Britain had developed AIDS and antibody testing had shown that 76 per cent of those who had had the concentrate were HIV positive.

In the United States, 80 hemophiliacs were known to have developed AIDS and the number of antibody positive people was proportionately great. In the British series, reported in the *British Medical Journal* in September, 1985, it was shown that 3 out of 36 sexual partners of antibody positive patients had also become positive. Three of the AIDS patients had died and a further 30 hemophiliac patients had pre-AIDS.

Although to cause AIDS in this way was a blunder of the first magnitude, it is hardly fair to blame the medical authorities in Britain and America. At the time Factor VIII and IX concentrates were first produced, AIDS had never been heard of. The same applies to the timing of the British decision to import concentrates from America. The question remains whether, once the fact of AIDS was known, suitable precautions were taken. In fact, no time was wasted. Since mid-1985, screening of all donated blood and blood products has virtually eliminated the risk of HIV transmission. Today, all blood products are most carefully checked for a range of viruses, including HIV and the hepatitis B virus, and plasma is treated to prevent the transmission of any known virus.

The situation was less satisfactory in France. There, at a meeting at ministerial level on 9 May 1985 the cabinet decided to defer acceptance of a screening test for blood proposed by the American pharmaceutical company Abbott. The Pasteur Institute was developing a similar test. A significant delay resulted during which French patients became infected with HIV. This unfortunate decision has led to the investigation of many prominent people including the then Prime Minister Laurent Fabius; Professor François Gros, secretary of the French Academy of Sciences; Georgina Dufoix, the then Minister of Social Affairs; Dr Claude Weisselberg, former adviser to the Health Secretariat; and Louie Schweitzer, chief executive of the Renault car manufacturer who was, at the time, chief of staff to the Prime Minister.

The AIDS causation blunders

The first general reports of AIDS came in a Morbidity and Mortality Report from the Centers for Disease Control (CDC) in Atlanta, Georgia, in June 1981. These unspectacular weekly reports, on trends in illness and causes of death, were useful to American doctors, keeping them up to date on disease trends and in monitoring epidemics and outbreaks of illness. But this report was different and sounded distinctly implausible.

It recorded a strange outbreak in Los Angeles of a very uncommon disease – a form of pneumonia caused by a little-known germ called *Pneumocystis carinii*. Two things about the report were remarkable. First, *Pneumocystis carinii* had always been believed to be of no medical importance whatsoever, and hardly ever caused harm. The second extraordinary thing about the report was that all five of the patients involved were homosexual men.

This innocent-seeming announcement by the CDC presaged a new disease and a new epidemic and posed a medical problem that was to grow to terrifying proportions and which would spread all over the world. It was to become a frightening puzzle which would tax the ingenuity and demand the dedicated labour of the best medical minds in the world. It was to involve medical scientists in a succession of new problems involving some of the most difficult aspects of medical science – studies into the intricacies of immunology and virology – and to

The BCG Tragedy

The Bacille Calmette-Guérin, is a French variant of the tubercle bacillus, obtained by repeatedly growing the organism to form a culture of colonies, and then regrowing one small sample of one of these. The aim is to produce a form that does not cause infection but that still prompts a protective immunological response in people who have not acquired such immunity naturally. Léon Calmette (1863–1933) and Camille Guérin, working at the Pasteur Institute, Paris, started the process in 1906 and for 13 years they patiently grew one subculture after another, until they had recultured the organism 231 times and were satisfied that the strain was safe. The vaccine, prepared from this strain, came into use in 1921. By 1928 it had been given to 116,000 children in France and was being widely used elsewhere, with a substantial reduction in the incidence of the disease.

Unfortunately, when a certain batch of the vaccine was given to 249 babies at Lubeck 67 of them died of acute tuberculosis. The vaccine was almost immediately withdrawn and there was widespread suspicion that the attenuated organisms were reverting to their original form. It was soon proved, however, that a terrible blunder had occurred in the preparation of these samples of the vaccine and that they had been accidentally contaminated with cultures of live and virulent tubercle bacilli. Germany and USA refused to approve BCG but it was widely adopted in Scandinavia where it considerably reduced the death rate from tuberculosis. Trials in Britain showed that it was safe and effective.

BCG is now established as a valuable method of conferring a measure of immunity on those who have not had the common, inapparent, primary infection and who are, in consequence susceptible to the disease. It reduces the likelihood of acquiring tuberculosis by about 80 per cent. Before considering BCG vaccination, a simple tuberculin test, the Heaf test, is used to determine the immune state of the individual.

* * * * *

Hand Washing

There is an old medical student joke that goes: surgeons wash their hands before they attend to the patient; physicians wash their hands afterwards. Surgeons, of course, have an elaborate ritual of scrubbing before donning sterile operating gowns and rubber gloves and are meticulous in the care they take to avoid contamination of any part that could come in contact with the operation site. If gloves are accidentally contaminated, they are immediately discarded and a new sterile pair put on. Some surgeons, anticipating contamination, will even wear two pairs so that the outer pair can be peeled off if soiled.

Away from the operating theatre, standards have not always been so high. In the wards, it has not been unknown for doctors to examine contaminated wounds and then wipe their hands on their white coats or handle the case notes. In the past, sloppy behaviour of this kind, while a cause of peer disapproval and raised eyebrows, never prompted more than mild censure. Sometimes, when a senior doctor has been the guilty party, his or her juniors have been able to do no more than glance, poker-faced, at one another. Usually, however, the immune system of the recipient of these iatrophoric germs (Greek *iatros*, a doctor; *phoreo*, to carry) has been able to cope and, in most cases, no great harm has been done.

involve the epidemiologists – specialists in the study of the spread of disease – in a detective story of unprecedented complexity and difficulty.

As more and more reports appeared of ever-larger numbers of men affected by this new disorder, it became apparent that homosexual men were also being attacked by another, quite different disease – Kaposi's sarcoma. Cases were occurring in New York and California, and the extraordinary thing about this outbreak was that Kaposi's sarcoma was also a disease which, for practical purposes, hardly ever affected young men of the age-group in which it was being reported. In addition to the Kaposi's sarcoma, four of these men had *Pneumocystis carinii* pneumonia. Other infective disorders, some common, some rare, were also affecting these men. These additional conditions included fungus infections, such as widespread thrush, extensive herpes infection and various unpleasant diseases that normally affected animals and birds rather than people. It was quickly apparent that the victims had little or no resistance to these infections. They were dying from severe infections caused by germs that were normally harmless. Clearly, something had happened to them to cause them to lose their normal immunity to infecting organisms.

Initial medical responses
Soon the CDC doctors formed a 'task force' to investigate the outbreak and to look into every aspect of the condition. And as the realization gradually dawned that this was no minor medical curiosity but a condition of grave importance and a problem of growing magnitude, CDC began to allocate more and more workers to the task force. Soon the reports indicated that the numbers of men affected were doubling every six months. In

the end, the problem came to be tackled by a larger force of investigatory and research medical scientists than has ever before in the history of medicine been mobilised for a single purpose. This was a measure of the concern which, rightly, came to be felt among the experts.

But what was the cause of this unheard-of loss of immunity? The doctors were familiar with cases in which, because of serious genetic disorders, immunity had never developed. But this was an acquired immune deficiency. So the condition came to be called the acquired immune deficiency syndrome or AIDS for short. (This is an acronym and should not be spelled 'Aids'.) The doctors were also familiar with a degree of immune deficiency from old age, from cancer or from heavy antibiotic usage, but none of these things applied here. It was a completely new situation.

Many theories were, of course, put forward to account for a severe degree of immune deficiency affecting, apparently, only homosexual men. Some of these theories were taken seriously and much time, energy and expense was devoted to their investigation. Instead of holding medical papers in a queue for months, articles and letters on AIDS were being printed at once – a striking indication of the strength of interest and the awareness of the importance of the subject.

One of the first things to be investigated was the lifestyle of AIDS victims. What was it that these unfortunate victims had in common? Information was soon available. Enquiries showed that AIDS cases were occurring in communities of homosexual men, whose lifestyle featured an exceptional amount of sexual activity – mainly homosexual but also bisexual – and characteristically involving large numbers of partners. Many would, as a matter of course, have sexual relations with more than 100 different partners in the course of a year. In addition, however, many of them were heroin addicts – often using the drug intravenously and often using the same needle repeatedly and communally.

Early theories

Another activity found to be almost universal in those with the disease was the use of 'poppers' – the inhalation of the volatile liquid amyl nitrite, originally intended for the treatment of angina pectoris, but commonly used in the gay community. Amyl nitrite comes in small, crushable glass vials, surrounded by gauze, and its effect is to produce an intense widening of most of the blood vessels of the body, so that the face flushes and the head throbs. The effect was used by the American gay community to enhance their orgasms and relax their anal orifices.

The liquid was readily available, being heavily advertised in magazines directed to the homosexual community, and was marketed ostensibly as a 'room deodoriser' or 'liquid incense'. Isobutyl nitrite, which has the same effects, was also being used. This compound has a smell vaguely reminiscent of sweaty socks and this compound was marketed under trade names such as 'Locker-room' and 'Aroma of men'.

The suggestion that inhalation of nitrites might be a factor in the causation of the syndrome excited a great deal of interest. Here, at last was a possible explanation of this extraordinary loss of immunity to infection and tumours. Here was a practice – the inhalation of an obviously powerful substance – which might well attack, and damage, the immune system. Investigation showed that over 80 per cent of the homosexual men attending sexually transmitted disease (STD) clinics in New

York, San Francisco and Atlanta admitted that they had inhaled amyl or isobutyl nitrites, and the data at the time strongly suggested that this practice was implicated in the immune deficiency. For a time it seemed that the problem was solved.

But there were one or two snags about this theory. The first one was that amyl nitrite had been inhaled by sufferers from angina pectoris for years and it had never been suggested before that it had affected their immune systems. Also, cases were beginning to appear in Britain – the first case of AIDS in Britain was reported in 1981 – and inhalation of nitrites was very much less common in Britain than in the United States. A report from one London STD clinic showed that only 30 per cent of the homosexual men had indulged in the practice. Back to square one.

The matter was becoming increasingly urgent. Many other explanations were put forward, considered and rejected. Marijuana smoking was one of the contenders and it was pointed out that this recreational drug had been shown to be able to interfere with the immune system. 'Angel dust', LSD, amphetamines and other drugs were considered. Again, it was suggested that seminal fluid, itself, might be responsible. This improbable theory was based on the fact that seminal fluid had been shown to contain powerful immunosuppressive substances and it was suggested that those who suffered bleeding during anal intercourse might acquire these substances. It was pointed out that some homosexual men greatly increased the risk of causing bleeding by wearing various spiky adornments on their penises.

One popular suggestion which, for a time, commanded a good deal of support was the idea that promiscuous homosexual people were exposed to so much infection – to so many different kinds of germs – that the capacity of their immune systems to resist disease was simply used up. It was, not unreasonably, supposed that there was a limit to the amount of resistance the body could mobilise and that people with the sort of lifestyle of the AIDS victims had reached their capacity. But this idea greatly underestimated the power and resources of the immune system and the theory was soon, apparently, disproved by laboratory tests. These showed that the AIDS victims still had normal numbers of the various cells that comprise the immune system. What was happening, apparently, was that some of these cells were not working properly. At that stage, even the most advanced workers in the field had only a fraction of the detailed knowledge of the immune system that doctors have today. There were subtle changes that were beyond their recognition at the time. So this theory was abandoned.

Other ideas were put forward. In April 1982, attention was drawn to the remarkable coincidence between the increase in the number of cases of AIDS and the ease with which cortisone-containing ointments could be bought over the counter. The doctor concerned pointed out that sales of these creams had increased enormously since they had become available and that they were widely used by male homosexuals to relieve the irritation and discomfort in the anal and genital regions resulting from sexual intercourse. Cortisone, he reminded the medical world, was a potent suppressor of the immune system and, used in this way, would be readily absorbed. Substantial doses could be acquired by passage through the thin skin of the penis, and the absorption would be aided by rubbing and mechanical trauma. This suggestion, like nearly all of the others, eventually passed into oblivion, but it was at least as plausible as many that were put forward.

Haitian immigrants and AIDS

Early in the American study it was noted that Haitian immigrants to the United States, many of them healthy, apparently heterosexual, men, seemed to be prone to develop the syndrome. The fate of ten of these immigrants was studied. All were said to be heterosexual and none of them had been using drugs. Six had tuberculosis, to which they seemed to have no resistance, but all of them responded well to standard methods of treatment. In addition to the tuberculosis, however, these unfortunate people developed several of the other manifestations of the condition, such as *Pneumocystis* pneumonia, thrush and a particularly unpleasant infection with a parasite called *Toxoplasma gondii*. Four of them developed brain abscesses from *T. gondii* and of the ten men in the study, six had died by the time the report on them was published.

These cases in Haitians, apparently differing in background from the earlier American cases, led people to speculate on whether this might provide a clue to the cause of AIDS. For a time, it seemed to be generally believed that Haiti was the origin of the disease and, inspired, no doubt, by tales of witchcraft and devil-raising on that 'mysterious' island, some imaginative theories were put forward. It was even suggested that the condition was caused by a virus which was originally an infection of domestic fowls and that it was first transmitted to man in the course of Voodoo ceremonies involving blood-letting and blood-smearing.

But there was a more plausible explanation. Towards the end of the 1970s Haiti had become a very popular vacation spot for gay people from America, and large numbers of American gay men had visited the island. It was not unreasonable to assume that the American visitors had transmitted the virus to Haitians.

This theory, of course, implied that AIDS could take a long time to show itself (had a long incubation period) and, since most of the Haitian patients appeared not to be gay, also suggested that the disease could spread to heterosexual people.

Theories such as the Voodoo idea do tend to catch the popular imagination especially among the group who found it impossible to escape the conviction that AIDS was God's latest round of punishment of the inhabitants of Sodom and Gomorrah. But, attractive though they may be to the righteous, such theories have to be tested and have to satisfy rigorous scientific criteria. And, unfortunately, when so tested, they failed to meet the facts.

After having to abandon the Haitian theory of origin, the epidemiologists began to look elsewhere and soon there was a general agreement that they were probably dealing with a Western form of a condition that had existed for a very long time in the developing countries. Their interest in this possibility was sharpened when their enquiries showed that, in the middle 1970s, there had been an upsurge of American interest in African culture and that this had led to a great increase in tourism in Africa.

The slim disease

So attention was drawn sharply to such records as could be obtained on the occurrence of similar diseases in Africa. These showed that cases of disease fitting precisely into the AIDS pattern – conditions such as that known as 'slim disease' – had been occurring in Central Africa as long ago as 1976, that is, well before the condition arose in the United States. Most of these reported cases occurred in Black Africans in Zaire, Rwanda, Gambia, and other central African countries, and there was now growing concern at the further risk of spread to other parts of the world from this source. What was most worrying was that AIDS occurred predominantly in people who engaged in highly promiscuous heterosexual activity. The implication was alarming. Here was a new source of AIDS infection, but of a type which was readily spread by heterosexual intercourse. A number of prostitutes working in Rwanda were examined. Nearly all of them showed some indications of AIDS or pre-AIDS and there was evidence that some of their consorts were also affected.

At last, however, it was becoming apparent that AIDS must be caused by an infection. In 1983 a French team at the Pasteur Institute, Paris, led by Dr Luc Montagnier, managed to isolate a virus from a patient with extensive lymph node enlargement and called it LAV (lymphadenopathy associated virus). About the same time, Dr Robert Gallo and his associates of the National Cancer Institute, Maryland, USA, demonstrated that a virus isolated from AIDS patients was the same virus. It was called HTLV-III. So now there were two names for the same organism and soon it became apparent that a new name was required. So the name human immunodeficiency virus (HIV) was chosen.

The discovery of the AIDS virus

AIDS was first reported in 1981, in Los Angeles and New York. As soon as its importance was appreciated, an immense research effort was mounted all over the world to discover the cause. In September 1983, Luc Montagnier, head of the Pasteur Institute in Paris sent to Robert Gallo, head of the tumour cell biology laboratory at the American National Cancer Institute, samples of the virus which had been isolated in his laboratory from an AIDS patient by Françoise Barré-Sinoussi, C. Cherman, F. Rey and others.

Seven months later Gallo held a press conference at which he announced he had discovered the cause of AIDS – a virus he called the human T cell leukaemia virus, group 3 or HTLV-III. He also announced that he had developed a blood test – an antigen-antibody reaction using the new virus as an antigen. Gallo was advised to patent the test and did so. In view of the huge number of people who would have to be tested for AIDS, this test was expected to become, and indeed proved to be, a major money-spinner although Gallo, as a government employee, had a strict limit placed on his own earnings from it.

In 1985 France sued the United States government, implying that Gallo had used the French virus for the test. For years, the Gallo team had been working on this class of human retroviruses and had described a similar virus, HTLV-I, in 1976. Workers in Gallo's laboratory, notably Mikulas Popovic, had solved the difficult problem of how to culture HTLV-III, so they were able to produce the large quantities needed for commercial exploitation of the test. Much other work of fundamental importance in immunology had come out of Gallo's laboratory. But efforts to trace the real origins of the virus now known to be the cause of AIDS and now called HIV, failed.

Gallo acknowledged the possibility that his virus may have arisen from contamination with LAV. Eventually, the dispute over royalties was settled when President Reagan and the French premier Jacques Chirac agreed that Luc Montagnier and Robert Gallo should share both the credit and the financial profits. But this was not the end of the affair. In 1989 the

Chicago Tribune published an article implying that Gallo had deprived the Pasteur Institute of credit for the discovery of the virus and concluded that his own claim of priority was based either on 'accident or theft'.

Investigation

An investigation was ordered and was undertaken by the American Office of Scientific Integrity. Its findings were published in September 1991. This body censured Gallo for self-aggrandizement and for detracting from the French achievement but concluded that his behaviour did not amount to misconduct. This report was criticized as whitewashing and pressure rose for a further enquiry by the Office of Research Integrity of the US Department of Health. Late in 1992 this body stated that in a research paper published in *Science* in 1984 Gallo had claimed that the French virus given him in 1983 had failed to grow in tissue culture. This, the enquiry had found, was 'knowingly false when written'. Gallo was accused of concealing information, of impeding the advancement of research and of abusing his senior status as a scientist. He was also accused of having a 'propensity to misrepresent and mislead in favour of his own research findings or hypotheses.'

These new findings overturned the previous verdict but the Office of Research Integrity, sensitive to criticism, drafted an appeals process to the Appeals Board of the Department of Health. This Board now instituted new legal standards for establishing misconduct. These required that there should be a genuine intent to deceive and that the consequences of the deception should be serious. Under the new more rigorous standards it was decided, and announced by the Office of Research Integrity, that it would not contest an appeal by

Gallo. Gallo claimed that he had been exonerated, but is at risk of investigation on the same charge by a Congress sub-committee. There have been allegations of a cover-up. The whole affair is an unpleasant blot on the fair name of science that has persisted for nearly a decade.

Chapter Four

Dangerous doctors

'Chevalier' Taylor's blinding career

Doctors are all too often not the source of a cure but the cause of disease or disability itself. Arrogance, presumption and plain foolishness have caused some doctors to persevere with theories and treatments that caused apalling damage and suffering to their patients. 'Chevalier' Taylor is a shining example of this. Two of the greatest musicians of all time, Johann Sebastian Bach and George Frederick Handel had the misfortune to meet and be treated by this medical blunderer.

John 'Chevalier' Taylor (1703–72) studied at St Thomas's Hospital, London, and travelled widely through England, Holland, and France as an itinerant oculist and eye surgeon. Taylor was medically qualified and had considerable skills as an operating surgeon, but was a bombastic self-advertiser and charlatan who, like others who have decided to treat medicine primarily as a source of income, enjoyed a remarkable lifestyle. At the time, ophthalmology was still in its infancy, but other, more reputable, surgeons were beginning to make real progress in treatment.

Taylor was one of the most successful surgical quacks in history and it is not, perhaps, surprising that he travelled so much. The crude operation he practiced for cataract – couching, in which the opaque lens was displaced within the eye – often gave brilliant immediate results which were followed by disastrous internal infection and inflammation. Infection within the eye, caused by the invariably contaminated couching needles, was invariably blinding and is still serious today, in spite of antibiotics. Largely because of his flamboyant lifestyle and advertisements, Taylor's fame spread to every country in Europe and his patients included many of the aristocracy and the royalty of Europe. Honours and degrees were showered upon him and he was welcomed into innumerable learned societies. He was 'Ophthalmiater' to the Pope, the Emperor and many Kings and Electors, whose names appeared on the title page of some of his books.

Taylor's victims
In spite of all his claims and assurances, Taylor's clinical results were, in fact, disastrous. Johann Sebastian Bach, on whom he operated, suffered agonies from repeated incisions into the eyes and from the use of mercury ointment and bleeding, but remained completely blind. Taylor's treatment undoubtedly hastened his death, but the 'surgeon' had the effrontery to claim that he had restored Bach's vision. George Frederick Handel became almost completely blind from cataract in 1743 and the self-styled 'Chevalier' Taylor operated on him also. Fortunately, Handel was spared infection from the unsterilized couching needle, but did not recover his sight. Taylor, of course, claimed afterwards that the operation had been a complete success. Sadly, within a few years there existed an effective and much safer method of treating cataract.

A treatise published in 1748 by the French surgeon Jacques Daviel started a revolution in ophthalmic surgery.

The great lexicographer Samuel Johnson wrote of Taylor: 'His career was an instance of how far impudence will carry ignorance.'

Horace Wells and the anaesthetic fiasco

At the end of 1844 the American dentist Horace Wells (1815–48) attended a public exhibition in Hartford Connecticut 'of the effects produced by inhaling Nitrous Oxide, Exhilarating or Laughing Gas.' This demonstration was given by an itinerant lecturer called Colton who had studied medicine but had never taken his degree. The handbills promised an interesting experience: 'The effect of the gas is to make those who inhale it either Laugh, Sing, Dance, Speak or Fight, and so forth, according to the leading trait of their character. Eight strong men are engaged to occupy the front seats to protect those under the influence of the gas from injuring themselves or others. This course is adopted that no apprehension of danger may be entertained. Probably no one will attempt to fight.'

Wells noticed that subjects under the influence of the gas, who were apt to fall about, showed no sign of pain when they struck themselves. One subject had gashed his leg deeply but felt nothing until the effects of the gas had worn off. At once it occurred to him that this gas offered a means of effecting painless dentistry. Having a troublesome molar, he persuaded Colton to go with him to his surgery where he inhaled some nitrous oxide and then had the tooth pulled by another dentist. He experienced no pain and decided to try it on his own patients. Within a month he had performed fifteen extractions under the gas, some of them with no experience of pain.

Realizing that this was a major advance in treatment Wells went to Boston with the intention of interesting the surgeons at the Massachusetts General Hospital. With the help of his former partner William Morton, now working in Boston, a demonstration was arranged in which Wells was to remove a tooth under nitrous oxide anaesthesia. Unfortunately, Wells's equipment – a silk bag full of the gas – was crude and he was inexperienced in administration and dosage. He was not aware that different patients required different amounts of the gas and he withdrew the bag too soon. It seemed at first as if the tooth had been removed without pain, but the patient, a boy, soon started roaring. Although he admitted that the pain had been less than usual, Wells's idea was officially rejected as a 'humbug affair'. Wells returned to Hartford, profoundly discouraged. The affair and his disappointment preyed on his mind and he became increasingly depressed.

The doctors were wrong. The following year Morton, who was aware of the reasons for Wells's failure and who had been investigating the properties of ether on the family dog and on himself, arranged to give his own demonstration at Massachusetts General. The news of this attempt quickly spread and the operating theatre was crowded with amused and sceptical spectators. The surgeon, Dr Warren, was in his usual formal morning clothes and the guards were ready to hold down the struggling patient. Morton was late and all presumed that he had lost his nerve. Dr Warren picked up his scalpel and silence descended. Turning to the spectators, he said, 'As Dr Morton has not arrived, I presume he is otherwise engaged.' At that juncture Morton hurried in. Dr Warren stepped back and politely indicated the patient. 'Well Sir,' he said, 'your patient is ready.'

The spectators watched in incredulous silence as the incision was made. The patient lay still, silent and uncomplaining, showing no signs of pain, and the operation was completed without incident. When he was finished Warren turned to the spectators.

'Gentlemen,' he said, 'this is no humbug.'

The subsequent widespread success of ether, rather than nitrous oxide, as an anaesthetic preyed heavily on Horace Wells's mind. He gave up dentistry and became a chloroform salesman. His practice of inhaling his wares soon led to addiction and in 1848 he was arrested for throwing sulphuric acid at two prostitutes on Broadway in New York. He was tried and sent to prison. Two days later he wrote a long letter to his family and the newspapers, and after attending a service in the prison chapel he used a razor blade to cut through the main artery in his left thigh and soon bled to death. Just a few days later a letter was received from the Paris Medical Society stating that the Society had recently officially credited Wells with the distinction of being the first to use general anaesthesia to perform painless surgery. Nitrous oxide soon came into widespread use as a pleasant and relatively safe anaesthetic agent – much safer, for instance, than chloroform – and is still in use today.

The addicted surgeon

William Stewart Halstead's name is known to every surgeon and to every student of medical history. He was born in 1852 and studied at Yale University where he was bored with study but turned out to be a star athlete. In his final year, however, he became interested in medicine and enrolled in the Columbia College of Physicians and Surgeons. He graduated in 1877 near the top of his class. After postgraduate training at Bellevue Hospital and the New York Hospital he spent two years training in Germany and Austria. He then returned to America where, after much experience in various New York hospitals he became a founding member of the faculty at John Hopkins Medical School, Baltimore.

He was a meticulous surgeon and a profound scholar of all things medical. He was also interested in his chief theatre nurse, Caroline Hampton. Caroline had sensitive skin and was much troubled by the irritating antiseptic chemicals that were in use at the time. So, in 1889, Halstead obtained some fine, thin rubber gloves for her to wear during operations. These were a great success. They were also easy to sterilize and it soon became apparent that rubber gloves could be a considerable advantage to the patient as well as to the staff. As a result it soon became routine for operating surgeons and their assistants to wear sterile gloves. It is to be supposed that Caroline was duly grateful; in any event, she married Halstead the following year.

During his long career at John Hopkins, Halstead was responsible for many other important advances. It was he who introduced the use of sterile surgical gowns, caps and masks to protect the patient from infection. In his time, these were invariably white; today they are usually green or pale blue to minimize glare. Halstead recognized that tissue should be handled with great gentleness and care and that all unnecessary blood loss should be avoided by clamping and tying off bleeding vessels. He became known as 'the bloodless surgeon'. His aseptic techniques were legendary and were widely influential. He invented several greatly improved operating instruments including fine artery forceps and a needle holder for curved stitching needles. He was also a notable originator of operations especially those for breast cancer and other cancers, hernia and overactivity of the thyroid gland.

What few people knew about this remarkable and successful man was that in the early 1880s, while experimenting on himself with the then new drug cocaine to produce local anaesthesia, Halstead had become profoundly addicted to the drug. Working with a colleague, Richard J. Hall, they had repeatedly injected each other with cocaine solutions of different strengths so as to find out what doses were needed for surgical anaesthesia. In this, they were highly successful and made a major contribution to surgery. Hundreds of thousands of patients benefitted from their discovery of nerve block anaesthesia. The advance exacted a heavy price from the researchers, however.

Halstead underwent several periods in hospital in an attempt to cure the addiction, but in vain. In desperation, he decided to try to displace cocaine with morphine. This quickly enabled him to give up cocaine but, inevitably, he became addicted to the alternative drug. In spite of this, his work record and the list of his achievements during the following period were both so impressive that most of his colleagues believed that he was no longer an addict, at the time of his appointment to Johns Hopkins Hospital.

Six months after his appointment, however, some of his associates discovered that he was still taking morphine. By then, he was so respected that the matter was kept secret. Halstead displayed almost incredible control in never allowing the addiction to get out of hand or to affect his work. This must have cost him dear. Even so, he was able to continue working at John Hopkins until his death in 1922, thirty-two years later. During the whole of that time he remained addicted to morphine.

The monkey gland affair

There must be some truth in the adage 'There's no fool like an old fool'. Throughout the ages elderly humans have longed for – and paid for – the secret of eternal youth. In every age, the quest has followed the technology or science of the time. First primitive magic, then alchemy, then crude pharmacology; and at each stage those concerned seem to have persuaded themselves that they were on to something good. In more recent times, the same process produced the conviction that medical science could do what all the efforts of the millennia could not – restore flagging bodily and sexual vigour. It may be significant that it has almost always been men who have applied for rejuvenation. Perhaps women have more sense.

Dr Serge Voronoff
The Russian-born physiologist and surgeon Dr Serge Voronoff (1866–1951) was Director of the Department of Experimental Surgery of the Collège de France. He was a flamboyant Parisian who, for a few years during the 1920s and early

1930s, achieved worldwide fame for achieving what appeared to be the greatest medical breakthrough of all time. It all started when Voronoff visited Cairo in 1898 and had the opportunity to examine some eunuchs – men who had been deliberately castrated at the age of six or seven. Voronoff was immensely struck by the appearance of these people whom he described as 'obese, with pendulous cheeks, smooth, hairless faces, developed breasts, enlarged pelves, flabby muscles, lethargic movements – all the signs so characteristic of the anaemic, feeble and flabby organism.' Their 'intellectual and moral characters' were, he thought, also in keeping with the physical signs and he decided that they were of slow intelligence, bad memory, and lacking in courage and enterprise. They were also, he thought, old before their time.

Fascinated, Voronoff took the opportunity to examine a large number of eunuchs and affirmed that these characteristics were common to them all. Quite reasonably, he concluded that all these effects were connected with the absence of the testicles. Since so many of the characteristics of eunuchs seemed to him to be similar to those of old age, it was but a short step to the idea that at least some of these effects should be reversible if the 'worn-out' testicle was replaced 'by one that was young and active'. By 1917, after years of experimentation on animals, Voronoff concluded that he had discovered how to achieve this desirable conclusion and embarked on the treatment of humans.

His operations were carried out simultaneously on the man and the ape, who were placed on separate tables in the same operating theatre. The ape was given a general anaesthetic with the volatile liquid ethyl chloride followed by chloroform, and the man a local anaesthetic. Both man and ape then had their scrotums, and the upper parts of their thighs, shaved, scrubbed with soap, hot water, and spirit and painted with iodine. The monkey's scrotum was then incised and one testicle removed. This was placed on a sterile pad and cut into six thin slices. In the meantime the other surgeon was opening the man's scrotum on one side and exposing the testicle which was then thoroughly scratched and roughened (scarified) so as to form a bed onto which the grafts would, hopefully, heal. Three testicular slices were then conveyed to the man, pressed into place and the layers of the scrotum closed with stitches. The same procedure was then done on the other side of the scrotum. While this was being done, the incision in the ape's scrotum was stitched and dressed.

Voronoff reported his results to medical journals and in a book called *Quarante-trois greffes du singe à l'homme,* translated into English under the title *Rejuvenation by grafting* and published in 1925. In this he claimed almost miraculous results and published many 'before and after' photographs purporting to show the results. Soon he was enjoying worldwide fame. Voronoff also claimed to be able, by such methods, to improve livestock, and the British Government was sufficiently impressed to set up a committee from the Ministry of Agriculture and Fisheries to report on his experiments. Their conclusions were carefully worded. They were optimistic about the eventual success of the method – most people were, at the time – but were unable to determine that there was any clear evidence of revival of sexual enthusiasm in old rams or for the claim of transmission of increased potency to the next generation. Quite rightly, they pointed out that Voronoff's trials were inadequately controlled and that his experimental conditions were unsatisfactory.

The general public were, however, all for it, and Voronoff decided to visit Britain in 1928. A public dinner was given for him and this was attended by many distinguished people including George Bernard Shaw, the Nobel Prize winner, Sir William Bragg, the Home Secretary Sir William Joyson-Hicks, and the Secretary to the Zoological Society of London. Voronoff also lectured at Cambridge, where he showed a film of his operation and 500 people turned up. Most believed that he was a brilliant pioneer of an important new technique. The next day *The Daily News* reported that some Harley Street surgeons were soon to begin offering the treatment. Voronoff tried to get a licence to perform the operation in Britain, but, largely because of Parliamentary pressure from anti-vivisectionists, this was refused.

In fact, Voronoff's first two monkey to human grafts had gone disastrously wrong; both patients had suffered severe wound infection and the grafts had had to be removed. Although many of his later patients had shown little ill effects, none enjoyed any benefit other than that produced by the powerful suggestion of the situation or possibly the short-term effects of the dose of testosterone from the donated tissue.

John R. Brinkley

Voronoff was an honourable, if misguided man. Others were less scrupulous, notably the Kansas surgeon John R. Brinkley. Encouraged by Voronoff's claims of success, Brinkley embarked on a wholesale campaign of testicular translocation, and was soon enjoying wide fame. The American authorities were less cautious than the British, and clearly thought that this was something too good to miss. Hundreds of prisoners in San Quentin jail were given grafts and were exposed to tacit pressure to report favourably. At the peak of his success, Brinkley was receiving 3,000 letters a day from prospective patients. For a time, few people had any doubts that the procedure was of genuine value. Unfortunately, Brinkley was a money-grubber who performed up to 50 operations a week and opened radio stations to advertise his wares. He became enormously wealthy, with many houses, a fleet of cars, two aeroplanes and a large yacht. When he finally came to justice, before Judge Burch of the Kansas Supreme Court, the judgement was colourful: '...the claimed result of which is that dotards having desire without capability may cease to sorrow as do those without hope. The defendant is not a quack of the common vulgar type. The gravamen of the complaint is that, being an empiric without moral sense, and having acted according to the ethical standards of an impostor, the defendant has perfected and organised charlatanism until it is capable of preying on human weakness, ignorance and credulity to an extent quite beyond the invention of the humble mountebank.' Brinkley lost his licence to practice, but immediately ran for Governor of Kansas, polling a respectable 183,278 votes – less than 34,000 below the winner.

Even before the truth of the matter was known, and while most still believed Voronoff's claims, the attack on him gradually mounted in ferocity, especially in Britain. An anti-Voronoff meeting was held in Caxton Hall, London, organized by the Duchess of Hamilton. Dean Inge preached a carefully worded sermon against monkey gland grafting in St Paul's Cathedral. Letters were written to *The Times* and other influential papers and critical pamphlets were published. There was, for a time, a body of opinion holding that, although the operation would succeed, it would have the effect of transmitting the characteristics of the donor monkey to future generations – a curious reversal of most people's understanding of Darwin's theory of evolution. It was also suggested that the operation could induce criminality in the patient. The British Thoroughbred Breeders Association discussed the matter and decided that no horse that had had the treatment should be allowed to have its name on the stud book.

By 1930 Voronoff was still generally popular and his operation was in great demand. Soon, however, scepticism began to grow, and proper scientific analysis began to show that such grafts could neither survive nor have the effects claimed for them. The hormone testosterone had been isolated from testicles in 1929, and extensive trials had shown that although it could maintain the secondary sexual characteristics of castrated animals and humans, it had no effect whatsoever on ageing. Around this time, the French veterinary surgeon Henri Velu published pioneering papers describing the microscopic events that followed grafts from a foreign donor and showed that such grafts attracted to themselves a massive attack by phagocytes and other defensive body cells. By the 1940s Peter Medawar's pioneering work on the immune system had showed that all such grafts would have been quickly rejected and destroyed.

Voronoff lived to be ridiculed, but bore it with dignity, and continued to study and write. At the age of sixty-five he fell in love with, and married, the beautiful twenty-one-year-old sister of the mistress of the King of Romania. King Carol awarded him a decoration. He died in 1951 at the age of eighty-five.

Brinkley's fortunes also declined. In 1938 he was described by the editor of an American medical journal as a quack, and made the mistake of suing for libel. This case brought the facts out into the open and Brinkley lost. Soon he was having a very hard time with litigious former patients, and had to pay out vast sums in damages. As a result, and owing $500,000 in unpaid tax, he declared himself bankrupt. He died of a heart attack in 1942 aged fifty-six.

The fall of Ferdinand Sauerbruch

The German surgeon, Ferdinand Sauerbruch was one of the greatest medical figures of the twentieth century, whose advances in the field of thoracic surgery (operations within the chest cavity) saved thousands of lives. Internationally revered before the Second World War, he worked in a succession of European capitals, and, at the Charité in Berlin, established a surgical unit whose reputation brought immense credit to his profession and his native country.

Such accomplishments, administrative as well as intellectual, required an immense and dominant will, and Sauerbruch's genius as a surgeon was complemented by his overbearing pride as an individual. Not that he was cold and unloveable – he inspired devotion in his colleagues not only for his skill with the knife but also for his essential humanity and concern for his patients – however he was an individual of rapidly fluctuating moods, whose kindness could freeze over in an instant should his authority be questioned. Then his ebullience turned to anger, and his terrible rages and icy scorn turned those around him to stone. It was this combination of reputation both professional and temperamental that made it difficult to contend with Sauerbruch when he lost his faculties and began to kill patients.

It was by then the post-war era; Berlin was divided, and

Sauerbruch, though in his seventies, was still heading the Charité, which fell in the Soviet-controlled sector, soon to become part of East Germany. Sauerbruch's name had been eclipsed by others in the West, but to Soviet surgeons and doctors, he was very much a hero. For political reasons it was important that Sauerbruch remain in the East, and the authorities showed themselves prepared to tolerate almost anything so that Sauerbruch might be seen to be co-operating with Communism. 'In the coming struggle of the proletariat, in the clash between socialism and capitalism, millions will lose their lives,' remarked one academic. 'In the face of this it is a trivial matter whether Sauerbruch kills a few dozen people on the operating table. We need the name of Sauerbruch.'

In 1904, aged twenty-seven, Sauerbruch had announced that he had discovered a way to perform surgery inside the chest cavity, a procedure then wholly revolutionary. Before, such operations had been impossible because low air pressure inside the lungs had meant that any surgical exposure of the thoracic cavity would result in its collapse and the death of the patient. Conducting experimental work under the most primitive conditions, Sauerbruch evolved his pressure differential technique, in which the patient was placed in a low pressure chamber. This permitted operations to be conducted on the lungs, heart and oesophagus and Sauerbruch was able to make great advances in the treatment of tuberculosis, and the removal of cancers and tumours. He had won over both disbelief and active opposition to make his discovery available to the public; there had also been deaths, and grim jokes were occasionally made to the effect that Sauerbruch's path to fame lay through his private cemetery.

Sauerbruch's father had died when Ferdinand was a child,

and he had been brought up by his grandfather, a shoemaker, in whose shop both Sauerbruch's mother and aunt worked. Later, in his entertaining if unreliable memoirs, Sauerbruch would recall watching his mother kneel at the feet of the clients, and how when he once admired a fine leather shoe, his grandfather had said to him, 'Those are the shoes one wears when one belongs.' The boy felt the family's lowly position acutely, and an early practical invention was a machine intended to save his mother from the humiliation of placing shoes on the feet of customers. On that occasion his grandfather laughed at him; but he remained inspired both by great practicality and his sense of social inferiority. In his efforts to transcend his origins, he was impatient of anything that he saw as petty, ideological, or intellectual opposition. He was filled with unshakeable confidence in his own abilities; this made him both a cheat (he attempted, and failed, to crib his way through early oral examinations in Greek by pretending he was deaf, and so needed to see the written text), and, in an age when surgeons depended on the patronage of the famous, the most honest of physicians. As an outsider he approached millionaires and kings with respectful assertiveness, was not afraid to tell the truth, and earned a reputation for blunt honesty.

The severity that served him well with the English nobility and the Swiss Rothschilds was not dropped when dealing with his colleagues; but rich company made him, in time, a frightful snob, and when dealing with those he came to perceive as lesser beings he could not distinguish honesty from disparagement. Reflecting on his reputation for rudeness and ill temper, Sauerbruch defended himself by saying that when he saw a great mistake being made he had simply neglected the hypocrisies of conventional courtesy; he would not say, 'My dear colleague, it strikes me that you have committed an error.' Instead, he explained, 'I would say "you idiot" or some similar expression of mild disapproval.' It was not, he argued, in the interests of the patient to beat about the bush.

Sauerbruch's mentor was the great German surgeon von Mikulicz, who was to him both father and teacher. It was the encouragement of von Mikulicz that rescued Sauerbruch from despair when the early experiments with pressure chamber thoracic surgery failed, and the first human patient died.

'We are not going to let the whims of an inanimate object rob us of the fruits of victory,' von Mikulicz told his protégé, who in a typical lapse of temperament had hidden himself in his room, weeping with frustration and anger.

'He was so kind and considerate,' recalled Sauerbruch, 'that he made me his slave for ever.' Von Mikulicz was a man of great energy, host of a famed intellectual salon, who was nonetheless always at the service of patients, and would not hesitate to operate in the early hours of the morning.

But it was only a few years before von Mikulicz began to suffer from strange lapses of skill, his powers failed, and he died of cancer. Sauerbruch found it excruciating to watch von Mikulicz's demise, and to see his 'eccentricities' of behaviour.

Sauerbruch's career had taken him from Breslau to Zurich, and thence to Berlin. He had travelled widely, had lectured across America, and since he was held in international respect could cross borders with ease during times of great political tension. It was this facility, the privilege of his profession, he was to claim, which had led to the German Kaiser employing him as a courier of secret messages to both the King of Bulgaria and the Sultan of Turkey during the First World War. Wherever he went, Sauerbruch caused ripples, and not only by his emotional excesses. From early years he was a heavy drinker and his appointment at Zurich was nearly jeopardized by his very public overconsumption of champagne; while waiting to hear news of his appointment he passed the time in his hotel finding out 'what kind of champagne a gentleman should drink.' It did his image no harm, however, that he should also be known as something of a philanderer, passionate in wooing, but chilly in conquest.

The one constant in Sauerbruch's character was similar to the quality he had so admired in von Mikulicz: his ability to subjugate all his immense energies to the service of his patients. In his devotion to the sick he was indifferent to class, nationality, or the patients' ability to pay. In fact, though he profited richly from prominent patients, he had little head for money, and his large household and impulsive acts of generosity constantly drained his resources. It was both flattering to him and a welcome moral obligation that the poor should seek him out because they had heard of his healing skill.

Throughout the First World War Sauerbruch had travelled between Zurich and the field hospitals near the frontline trenches. The use of artillery in modern warfare caused a variety of injuries necessitating the amputation of arms or legs, and another of the surgeon's contributions was the invention of an artificial hand, which could employ the muscles left in a truncated stump.

By the Second World War he was ensconced at the Charité, where he continued operating on the injured even as the Russians shelled the city to rubble. In April 1945, the Russians entered the underground bunker which was by then serving as an operating theatre. A nervous Russian soldier accidentally discharged a few rounds into the floor, and one of these hit a nurse in the foot. Otherwise, the transition from Nazi to Soviet control of the hospital was a peaceful affair.

From the moment the Soviets assumed control of the hospital, they sought out Sauerbruch, coming as patients, or to offer him homage in money or goods. War had much reduced his circumstances, and their gifts of tinned food and wine were welcomed by his wife and housekeeper, who had also struggled to bring home to the great man any provision they could now that he was quite indigent. Whereas most other private dwellings were looted, and female occupants raped, a notice was posted outside Sauerbruch's house, notifying Soviet soldiers that this was the residence of the 'great surgeon' – it thus escaped being pillaged. And, quite extraordinarily, Sauerbruch was given a car; the personal gift of General Kotikov.

The Americans were more curious as to Sauerbruch's relations with the Nazis, and had him removed from the Municipal Public Health Board. But the Soviets helped him to rebuild and re-equip the Charité and let him employ the assistants he desired.

This last liberty was of paramount importance to Sauerbruch. He was seventy-two, and his operating procedure had long depended upon the support of a highly disciplined team who would conduct all preliminary work on a patient and make the initial incisions, leaving him to concentrate his powers solely on the excision, or restorative work. When closing up a wound, he might make the initial sutures, but an assistant would generally complete the job. Such a procedure enabled him to operate on a continuous line of patients. The regime that concentrated his efforts on his skill with the knife extended beyond the hospital. His wife, housekeeper, and chauffeur all adhered to a strict timetable so that Sauerbruch's routine was undisturbed and he might be at his best with the knife. The war had taken his long-established assistants from him; new assistants did not stay long. Either he sacked them or they could not tolerate his temper.

Sauerbruch's first appointment was a German surgeon, Max Madlener, a first-rate physician in his late forties. Madlener was known to have served with the SS. Though the appointment was not opposed, it was noted. Complaints were made by the Americans, and the matter came to the attention of Doctor Friedrich Hall, the new supervisor for medical faculties in East Berlin. Hall was a young German neurologist who had been captured by the Soviet army, and returned to Germany to all appearances a committed Communist. He retained, though, a consideration for individual life that was not wholly compatible with the absolute ideology of his new masters.

Hall visited Sauerbruch, who was living and working in impoverished circumstances. When he raised the matter of Madlener he was accused of being one of many who were attempting to politicize the surgeon's work. The eminent man was coherent, if irate, throughout the majority of the interview, but as a neurologist Hall could not help but note that towards the end of their talk Sauerbruch began to repeat himself, that his sentences remained incomplete, that he forgot names, and that he referred to the dead as if they still lived and he might have seen them only the day before.

Hall knew that Sauerbruch had a reputation for intellectual vigour. He ascribed such incongruities to fatigue and age, but later, in considering the state of the surgeon – his untidiness and preoccupation – he began to worry about his mental health. Then, by chance, some tapes of Sauerbruch lecturing before the war were recovered from the rubble of Berlin. When he heard these, Hall concluded that there was such a marked deterioration in the surgeon that it was possible even to make a diagnosis; that Sauerbruch's incoherence was a symptom of cerebral sclerosis, which made him as dangerous with the knife as a drunk might be.

In fact, unknown to Hall, Sauerbruch had already been involved in at least one unnecessary death. In May 1946, Sauerbruch had operated on Hans Greif, a thirty-nine-year-old German actor who had fled to Russia to become the German voice of Radio Moscow. Greif had been operated on for a hernia, and in the course of the operation Sauerbruch had wounded an arterial blood vessel, applied clamps and trapped a branch of the femoral artery. Greif died of a hemorrhage the next day.

It was an uncharacteristically slapdash piece of work by the surgeon. Those close to Sauerbruch were convinced that he recognized that his powers were failing, and interpreted his employment of Madlener as an indication that he was looking for a disciple and successor. The younger man's loyalty to Sauerbruch was to prove a frustration to the authorities. When Hall raised the issue of Sauerbruch with his superiors, he was told that the surgeon's condition was known about, but that the appointment of Madlener was a sure sign of Sauerbruch's self-knowledge; he would step down of his own accord.

This did not happen. In the autumn of 1948, Hall discovered that Karl Stompfe, a respected surgeon, had resigned the position of First Resident at the Charité after Sauerbruch had physically assaulted him. Stompfe had pointed out to Sauerbruch that he was operating with dirty hands; this had precipitated a furious tirade about treachery. Hall, now very concerned, visited Sauerbruch once more. He found him sitting blank-faced in his office. Hall attempted to broach the subject of Stompfe, but in the middle of their conversation, the surgeon was summoned by Madlener to attend to a cerebral tumour. Within minutes he returned to his office clutching the malignant growth in his hand. The fingers, he said to Madlener, made the best surgical tools; he had wrenched off the tumour, and the patient died two days later.

It occurred to Hall that he should enquire of the pathology department at the Charité about the causes of unexpected deaths among the hospital's patients. He found Rossle, the professor of pathology, distinctly reticent; but it was true, he admitted, that there was a problem with Sauerbruch, which many knew about, but for reasons of personal or political loyalty were unable to act on. Understanding from this that many people were dying under the surgeon's knife, Hall requested of his superiors that Sauerbruch be removed immediately. His cerebral sclerosis was untreatable. It was then that he met with ideological opposition; it would be too embarrassing if Sauerbruch were to be sacked, since questions would inevitably be raised in the West. If he were to go, he must go of his own accord.

In April of 1949, there was further public evidence of Sauerbruch's deterioration, when he flew into a rage at his de-Nazification hearing. That Sauerbruch had despised the Nazis was well known, and he had publicly derided Hitler. But he was a patriot, and proud of his achievements and he had, like many others, accepted tainted honours and property that had been confiscated from Jews. There was little prospect of the tribunal finding against him, but he took offence at their obligatory questions, threatened to vomit over all present, and walked out declaring he was going home.

As travel links were restored throughout Europe, Sauerbruch became once again in demand for private consultations, and could be found wandering, quite bewildered and lost, around major airports. Late in 1949, in the presence of Madlener, Sauerbruch operated on a boy suffering from cancer of the stomach. Obliged to remove part of the intestine, he sutured it and the stomach separately. The boy died.

Hall had by now acquired the autopsy records from the Charité pathology clinic, which confirmed his worst fears. He confronted Madlener, who admitted that he was aware of the problem; he refused, however, to accede to Hall's request that he confront Sauerbruch. Madlener would have been Sauerbruch's successor, but his sense of gratitude to Sauerbruch was such that he regarded any discussion about usurping his master as wholly disloyal. He did, however, suggest that the authorities might avoid a confrontation by simply retiring all professors at the Charité over the age of seventy. Hall's superiors agreed, and Madlener broke the news about the ruling to Sauerbruch, making it seem as impersonal as possible. The great surgeon was furious and suspicious in equal measure. An honourable resignation, on a preferential pension, would have been the correct decision. But Sauerbruch continued as before.

His assistants attempted to shield acute patients from him, but inevitably there were fatalities. The authorities tried to evade responsibility, blaming Madlener for failing to intervene and again instructing him that he should assume control of the hospital. Again Madlener refused. Professor Rossle, another old colleague of Sauerbruch's, now retired as head of the pathology unit of the Charité, approached the surgeon who became violent and accused Rossle of trying to ruin him.

Finally, Paul Wandel and Theodor Brugsch, the Minister for People's Education, and the former director of the first medical clinic at the Charité, respectively, invited Sauerbruch to drinks and supper; and in social circumstances that inhibited his rage, appealed to his pride, saying that they were concerned for his sake that he resign before suffering the humiliation of being sacked. It was, they argued, inconceivable that he should work for those who had no respect for him, and did not want his services.

On 3 December 1949, Wandel and Brugsch waited in Wandel's office, anxiously wondering whether Sauerbruch would still come and meet them, as had been agreed, and formally tender his resignation. The surgeon came; but he did not resign without strife. Instead, he had to be asked such questions as, 'Do you wish to begin your retirement?' and, 'Are we to understand that you are making this step of your own free will?' To these he mumbled replies; then followed a tantrum, and Sauerbruch stormed out.

He continued to visit the clinic, until the staff complained and he arrived one day to find his office door locked. Though much impoverished, he also refused the generous settlement offered in addition to his pension. To general horror, he announced that he would work at a private clinic in Grunewald, whose owner was unaware of Sauerbruch's condition, and thought that his name would ensure the good reputation and profit of the enterprise.

But such had been Sauerbruch's reputation for generosity that the clinic was inundated by the old and poor who traced Sauerbruch through the Charité. Previously, he had had the resources of the state at his disposal, but his new employer had limited finances for such philanthropy. Moreover, it became quickly evident that the surgeon had not been sacked because of professional jealousy, as he was now claiming. When not promising to relieve the tired masses who came to the door, he sat in silence, looking lost, in a dilapidated office. It was decided that he could not be allowed to operate, but should be retained as a consultant.

In their efforts to find him, the sick besieged his decaying, cold house. His wife disconnected the doorbell. When Sauerbruch stumbled across the needy on his doorstep, he still instructed them to come to him at the clinic. Often he told his housekeeper to give them money. There was no money, and she herself spent her savings to maintain the surgeon.

Hearing that Sauerbruch was so impoverished, a publisher who had once served as an orderly to him suggested that he should write his memoirs. These were to be ghosted by Hans Rudolf Berndorff. Despatched to negotiate a contract, Berndorff was informed that Sauerbruch was attending a conference at Wiesbaden. Sauerbruch told Berndorff that he was staying in a fine hotel; Berndorff found him in a hospital room, where he had been placed by the conference organizers. He was quite incoherent, willingly signed a contract scribbled on a scrap of paper, and offered to remove a node he had spotted on the writer's hand. The memoirs proved a convoluted business. Sauerbruch would reminisce to various despairing secretaries, and Berndorff then endeavoured to introduce a vein of consistency into the mixture of touching recollection, professorial observation and Munchausen-like lies.

Among the most preposterous – but compelling – of his tall stories was that concerning General Ludendorff, Germany's supreme military commander in the First World War. Sauerbruch claimed that he had diagnosed Ludendorff as having suffered for many years from a thyroid complication. Surmising that this condition might have affected his leadership during the conflict, Ludendorff agreed to surgery only on condition that it was performed without anaesthetic. In this way he did penance for losing the war. Sauerbruch also claimed to have operated on Lenin, Mussolini, the King of England (he could not be more specific), and Count Hindenburg.

Sauerbruch could not forsake his knife. In 1950, prevented from operating at the Grunewald clinic, he undertook surgery in the cold squalor of his own home. He had no anaesthetic, and his instruments were filthy. His wife and housekeeper put the patients in the family beds, and tried to console them. Rumours of macabre happenings reached the authorities, who repeatedly requested of Sauerbruch's wife that she stop him; they themselves would take no action.

But Margot Sauerbruch, herself a doctor, was obliged to work full time in order to make ends meet. The moment she left the house, her husband would begin operating once more. His frustrations now showed themselves in obsessive tics and phrases. He scanned all those he met for nodes, cysts and varicose veins, and instead of exchanging pleasantries he would seize greedily at any growth, real or imagined, and say, 'I must operate on that. I'll do it at once.' His compulsion to practice was greater even than his once renowned spirit of romance. Taken by his publisher to visit Erna Hanfstaengl, an old flame with whom he had conducted a passionate and scandalous romance, he took her withered hand and said he must immediately remove the brown spots from it.

In April 1951, Sauerbruch operated on a middle-aged woman who in her youth had been a patient of his, and had never ceased to revere him. She could not afford a private hospital, and Sauerbruch conducted surgery without anaesthetic, in his drawing room, making an eight-inch incision in her throat to remove a cancerous growth. She was put in Sauerbruch's room, where she deteriorated, dying some months later in hospital, in excruciating pain. She did not blame the surgeon.

Sauerbruch was by then already dead. When his wife had this last patient removed from the house, her neck weeping pus, the authorities were compelled to ban him from seeing any patients whatsoever. This would have proved impossible to enforce without physical restraint. But, thwarted from immediately diverting himself with others, Sauerbruch's sclerotic compulsion turned suddenly inwards. He had taken to getting in his car, and ordering his chauffeur to drive to his places of former employment. Instead, the chauffeur would drive Sauerbruch aimlessly around the city and out into the country, since the movement seemed to comfort his master.

On a May afternoon, they were driving through farmland green with spring crops, when Sauerbruch sighted a farmer, walking slowly across a field adjacent to the road. Ordering his chauffeur to stop, Sauerbruch leapt from the car, jumped over the hedge and set off across the mud and shoots of wheat, shouting at the farmer that he was a fool, an utter fool. The surgeon had barely caught up with the farmer when he collapsed, clutching his stomach in great pain. He was carried back to the car, and taken to hospital where he died on 2 July 1951.

The first blood transfusions

The first blood transfusions were carried out, without the consent of the patients, in the 1880s by Dr Braxton Hicks, a gynaecologist at Guy's Hospital in London. He thought transfusion might, in theory, be possible and tried it on four patients, using sodium phosphate as a possible anticoagulant. Needless to say, he had at that stage not the faintest idea about blood groups and all four patients died. There were no ethical research committees, and no question of litigation against him arose.

* * * * *

Women doctors

The Victorians were petrified at the prospect of women entering the medical profession as anything other than nurses. The first female doctor was an imposter, the extraordinary Dr James Barrie, who passed herself off as a man. She qualified in Edinburgh in 1812 and subsequently pursued a distinguished but tempestuous career in the army, even fighting a duel. She ultimately rose to be Director General of Hospitals, a rank equivalent to that of a major-general. Her deception was not discovered until her death, aged seventy. A charwoman who laid out her corpse discovered to her shock that Barrie was a woman, and even possessed stretch marks on her lower abdomen which indicated that she had, at some point in her life, given birth to a child.

Misdiagnosis today

A recent survey by researchers at Sheffield University in England found that doctors are failing to alert coroners' courts to scores of deaths under suspicious circumstances because of their inability to diagnose the cause of death. Only two out of three cases requiring referral were correctly identified. Out of sixteen case histories presented to 200 doctors, the number of correct answers ranged from only three to eleven. The greatest cause for worry was that deaths due to medical treatment – iatrogenically induced deaths – were the least often correctly identified. In fact, doctors opted not to refer as suspicious deaths which had occurred within twenty-four hours of admission to a hospital or an operation. In America, a 1983 study published in the Journal of the American Medical Association studied 100 consecutive cases in which autopsies had conclusively revealed that the cause of death was a heart attack. They were shocked to discover that in only 53 per cent of the cases had the doctors present at the death correctly diagnosed the cause of it. Nearly half of all deaths from heart attack were going undiagnosed, or being blamed on something else, and nearly half the cases were managed by cardiologists – so-called experts in the field of heart disease. A nationwide survey compared 1,800 diagnoses made on living patients with the subsequent revelations of the autopsy. They found an error rate of nearly 20 per cent, and it was estimated that about half of those misdiagnoses led directly to the patients' deaths.

The toxin doctor

Dr Ernst Hofstadter was nothing if not impressive. A little below average height and in his mid-fifties, he was slim, spry, and always immaculately dressed. His collars were as snow, his bow ties models of perfection, his cuff links discreet but obviously very expensive. Each day a perfect fresh carnation or rose adorned his lapel. His beard was small and neatly trimmed; his skin clear and sallowish; his accent cultivated, middle-European and very authoritative.

His manner was deeply courteous, attentive, sympathetic; above all, understanding. His patients – all private – were never in any doubt that they were getting their money's worth.

Dr Hofstadter had a degree from an obscure Middle Eastern medical school and had had some difficulty in persuading the General Medical Council to recognize his qualifications, but in the end had succeeded. Although possessing only a basic registrable qualification Hofstadter called himself a specialist. His subject was a disease known as ileo-jejunal toxosis. This condition did not feature in any of the orthodox medical textbooks but had been described at length in a popular paperback book Hofstadter had written some years before. The book, *The Toxic Bowel Syndrome*, was now in its 11th printing and continued to sell well. The royalties (Hofstadter got 15 per cent of the cover price of every copy sold) were substantial but they were nothing to the income generated by the resulting large numbers of patients who, as a result of reading the book, decided to consult him.

The main reason for this enthusiastic response was that Hofstadter's book attributed such a wide range of symptoms to the disease ileo-jejunal toxosis, and related these symptoms so circumstantially to items likely to be found in almost every person's diet, that nearly every one who read the book was convinced that he or she had the disease. Hofstadter was careful not to recommend himself in the book; indeed, he went so far as to state that self-advertising of that kind was abhorrent and was rightly condemned by the GMC. He was, however, quite clear about his motive in writing the book. This was solely to save the Government the millions of pounds currently being wasted in the National Health Service through their unfathomable refusal to adopt his treatment.

On the exact details of this treatment, he was strangely vague. There was, however, a clear implication that the detoxification process, to be effective, called for the skilled management of a specialist who had made a thorough study of the condition. Dr Hofstadter's name was in the phone book, and his charming secretary always responded so positively and welcomingly to any enquiries, that few who called failed to get an appointment to see the doctor.

Dr Hofstadter had a no-lose technique. If the patient recovered – and most patients do, with or without treatment – the doctor took the credit. If they did not, the case was one of particular difficulty and of absorbing interest to the doctor and called for extended therapy. This would inevitably be successful, but one would have to recognize that some forms of the disorder took quite a time to resolve. Patience was necessary. The doctor's diagnostic methods were very expensive but most impressive. They involved CT scans and MRI imaging and a range of laboratory tests requiring the removal of an alarming quantity of blood. Sometimes, to clear up a slight diagnostic ambiguity, he would resort to the use of a diamond pendulum which he would swing, for minutes at a time, over the patient's naked abdomen. His head-to-toe clinical examinations were careful, comprehensive and time-consuming and no orifice was left unexplored. Throughout, his expression remained impassively watchful and it was clear that he would allow no emotion, either of surprise or of satisfaction to disturb his admirably detached gravitas. His explanations were couched in elaborate terminology, expressed always with a deeply flattering confidence in the patient's power of comprehension.

Dr Hofstadter was a virtuoso in the exploitation of the placebo effect. Almost all whom he treated with his expensive intravenous detoxification agent (formulated uniquely for each patient) came back to tell him how much better they felt. He was also a virtuoso in the art of positive transference. Many of his lady patients believed themselves in love with him, and some of the men thought they perceived amorous possibilities. The net effect was that once a patient had come under his spell, that person was likely to remain his patient indefinitely.

Over the years, Dr Hofstadter's practice, and his bank balance, grew exponentially. He became rich and widely appreciated – except by the medical profession. Eventually he came to interpret his success as a clear indication that his theories must be true. At first, this raised the difficulty that the terms in which he habitually expressed his theories were meaningless. Pseudo-scientific jargon does not actually convey anything. 'Ileo-jejunal' simply means 'pertaining to the small intestine' and 'toxosis', if it means anything at all, just means 'a state of poisoning'. But if one uses a phrase thousands of times, it is apt to acquire some kind of meaning and Dr Hofstadter became an ardent believer.

He began to write articles for the *British Medical Journal* full of statistically impeccable proofs of the efficacy of his methods. These were politely returned as being unsuitable for publication. He wrote a thesis for a Doctorate, but no university would countenance it. Eventually, he decided that if the Establishment was going to ignore him he would simply have to found his own medical journal. This turned out to be rather more expensive than he had expected, and in more ways than one. The *Journal of Dietary Assimilative Toxicology*, edited, and largely written, by E. Hofstadter, got off to an excellent start. Numerous papers were received, mainly from people who could not get published elsewhere. Unfortunately Dr Hofstadter had not, for years, been exposed to scientific medicine and was in no position to adjudicate on the merits of these papers. As a result he rejected the more orthodox and, so as not to appear to be the sole author, published those that most closely conformed to his own ideas.

After four monthly issues, distributed free to thousands of doctors but containing a conspicuous registration and order form, the ingenious doctor was forced to tot up his losses. Only about a dozen people had taken out subscriptions and not even the most outré of the alternative medicine firms would advertise in the journal. The bills for office overheads, printing and distribution were ruinous. As he had had to devote his full time to the new journal there was no income from his practice. A hasty calculation indicated that he would be ruined within a year. Reluctantly, he decided to cut his losses and close down.

Unfortunately, although most doctors had simply chucked Dr Hofstadter's journal into the waste bin, many had taken the trouble to read it. Some of these, aware that the theories of toxic absorption from the bowel had been denounced as arrant nonsense half a century earlier, were prompted to condemn the journal in the correspondence pages of the reputable medical press. These letters were published without editorial comment and attracted the attention of two investigative journalists, ever on the lookout for a juicy story. Dr Hofstadter, approached by these men, was indiscreet enough to boast about the size of his practice.

The whole business then became public knowledge and soon the doctor's telephone ceased to ring. Not long afterwards Dr Hofstadter felt the call of his native land and left these shores for ever. He did so with a thoughtful expression, pondering intently on the question of whether there might be a better alternative to hormone replacement therapy for the mature woman ...

The moral of this entirely fictitious tale, as the attentive reader will have perceived, is that there is much to be said for whitewash so long as it doesn't make the holes in the fence too conspicuous.

Defensive medicine

From fear of litigation arises the ludicrous prospect of defensive medicine, already widely practiced in America, whereby doctors will charge for doing little or nothing, excessively employing all-purpose prophylactic drugs, like antibiotics, in unnecessary circumstances, or frantically advise expensive tests to cover themselves. In 1977, the American Medical Association conducted a survey which showed that 75 per cent of their members took X-rays and other tests unnecessarily in order to protect themselves. In 1984, it was estimated that defensive medicine was adding $15.1 billion to the nation's annual medical bill. Defensive medicine probably accounts for Caesarean section being four times more common in America than elsewhere; the obstetrician will choose this course if normal delivery looks even remotely difficult. The danger of causing brain damage to the child is an expensive risk.

* * * * *

Surprising mortality rates

In the first few weeks of 1976, physicians in Los Angeles county went on a work-to-rule, and withheld all but emergency services. As a consequence, 'elective' surgery (surgery which is non-essential but which the patient, after taking advice from his doctor, 'elects' to have) was stopped. Despite alarmist reports in local newspapers about what a terrible effect this would have on the population's health, subsequent examination of the data showed that during this period, when non-essential surgery and medical treatment ground to a halt, there was a fall in the mortality rate, which picked up to normal proportions when doctors went back to business. The same happened in Israel in 1973, when the nation's death rate dropped by a staggering 50 per cent during a surgeons' strike, and again in Brazil, where a strike by doctors led to a 35 per cent decline in the rate of mortality.

The problem of addicted doctors

In America, a recent report in the *Medical Tribune* stated that of the doctors in practice, between 22,600 and 36,600 were recovering alcoholics, or on the path to alcoholism, and that drug addiction was between thirty and a hundred times more prevalent among doctors than among the general public. In fact, a 1975 report revealed that one in six known drug addicts in the USA, Britain, the Netherlands, France, and Germany was a doctor, and other statistics claimed that up to 13 per cent of American doctors would have an addiction problem in the course of their careers; an article in Medical Economics in 1985 showed that abuse of prescription drugs was four times the national average among doctors and that their cocaine habits had increased tenfold in the previous five years. Studies of drug-taking in American medical schools showed that the nation lost the equivalent of seven graduating classes each year to drug addiction, alcoholism, and suicide.

* * * * *

Misread X-rays

Some 43 million Americans a year are having their X-rays misread and their illnesses consequently misdiagnosed or undiagnosed. Those are the conclusions drawn from research by the American Leonard Berlin, MD. Despite advanced equipment, good facilities and specialized teaching, he found that radiologists working at an eminent university disagreed on the interpretation of chest X-rays over half the time, and made potentially significant errors over 40 per cent of the time. Berlin blamed these figures on the haste with which X-rays were examined. Through greed, defensive medicine, or the belief that no consultation is complete without the use of technology, billions of unnecessary X-rays are taken, and the radiologist in a hospital has only five or ten minutes for each patient.

Therapeutic beneficence

Because of their training, we presume that doctors are unlikely to suffer from these sorts of human problems. For centuries, the security of the doctor-patient relationship has been passed on this premise, sustained by the paternal role of physicians. Hippocrates, the Greek physician, whose code is still symbolically that of the modern medical profession, wrote that the physician should: 'Declare the past, diagnose the present, foretell the future; practice these acts. As to disease, make a habit of two things – to help, or, at least, to do no harm.'

Hippocrates also laid down specific advice aimed at preserving the priestly status of the physician, and in an essay entitled 'Decorum' he sketched out a bedside manner in which the emphasis is firmly on giving as little away to the patient as possible; these are instructions for a performance: 'On entering, bear in mind your manner of sitting, reserve, arrangement of dress, decisive utterance, brevity of speech, composure, bedside manners, care, replies to objections, calm self-control to meet the troubles that occur ... Perform all this calmly and adroitly, concealing most things from the patient while you are attending him. Give necessary orders with cheerfulness ... turning his attention away from what is being done to him; sometimes reprove sharply and emphatically and sometimes comfort with solicitude and attention, revealing nothing of the patient's future or past condition ... For many patients through this cause matters have taken a turn for the worse, I mean by the declaration I have mentioned of what is present, or by a forecast of what is to come.

Physicians were also discouraged from undertaking to treat potentially fatal cases; their position depended upon success, and it was not good publicity for the profession to have one's patients dropping dead. Until the introduction, after the Second World War, of the notion of informed consent in the USA, much was habitually withheld from patients. Doctors would wish to conceal their doubt, and, when they did know what was happening, argued that the psychological effects of knowing the truth might be detrimental to the patient's chances of recovery. A doctor's right to judge what it is best for his or her patients to know, and to lie accordingly, is known as 'therapeutic beneficence'.

'Therapeutic beneficence' has had many passionate advocates. Henri de Mondeville, a fourteenth-century surgeon, teacher of anatomy, and influential pioneer in the field of medical ethics, urged his pupils to 'promise a cure to every patient but ... tell the friends or parents if there is any danger.'

De Mondeville placed great faith in the power of human optimism, and also the curative effects of ambition. The surgeon was not to be afraid to lie if it benefits the patient, he wrote: 'For example, if a canon is sick, tell him that his bishop has just died; the hope of succeeding him should bring about a rapid cure ...'

Patients were to be entirely submissive and 'obey their surgeons in everything'. Surgeons were entitled to exact obedience by threatening their patients with dire consequences and exaggerating information with the express purpose of terrifying them; any difficult patients were to be refused treatment as their opposition would reflect badly on one.

Over three hundred years later, de Mondeville's principles were reiterated by Benjamin Rush, a hugely knowledgeable physician who lectured on medical ethics and was known as 'the American Hippocrates'. Rush said that physicians should 'yield to their patients in matters of little consequence, but maintain an inflexible authority over them in matters that are essential to life... the obedience of a patient to the prescriptions of his physician should be prompt, strict, and universal. He should never oppose his own inclinations nor judgement to the advice of the physician.'

This was in an age when, as Voltaire said, medicine was principally a matter of 'amusing the patient while nature cures the disease', and the quack and the accepted doctor were largely indistinguishable. In the absence of true knowledge about the origins of even the most minor complaints, it was essential that the appearance of medical authority was maintained. To preserve their mystique and connection with the priestly status enjoyed by ancient physicians, doctors persevered in speaking Latin in front of their patients.

In the nineteenth century, the proliferating medical profession was still largely useless, and depended increasingly upon the accoutrements of respectability. Oliver Wendell Holmes, an American physician and man of letters, put it succinctly when he wrote that, to be successful, the physician needed 'a top hat to give authority, a paunch for dignity and balance and piles to cause an anxious, caring expression'. Holmes also famously wrote as late as 1883 that 'if the whole materia medica as now used could be sunk to the bottom of the sea, it would be all the better for mankind and the worse for the fishes'.

With medicine still a matter of speculation, the patient had no legal recourse for ill-treatment, although it was quite common for doctors to be accused of fathering any unwanted children in their district of practice. If a patient died, as often happened, there was no question of suing the physician.

Of course, as medicine evolved, there were doctors who

wished to bring to the public the practical benefits of new knowledge, but whereas a doctor would not be struck off the Medical Register (begun in 1845) if effectively killing patients, the Victorian doctor was strongly advised to avoid releasing information on such areas of popular ignorance as birth control; there were things the public should not know about. Doctors sought to protect their status by casting themselves as defenders of moral standards, and the new medical bodies formed in this period sought to incorporate, and give moral and legal authority to that paternal right of 'therapeutic beneficence' which the doctor had hitherto exercised at his discretion.

In 1887 Arthur Allbutt, a consultant physician in Leeds, wrote a little book called *The Wife's Handbook*. It was principally about childcare, but there was a highly informative concluding chapter entitled 'How to Prevent Conception', in which Allbutt sought to discredit some of the useless contraceptive methods widely practiced. Among these was the belief that the wife had only to sit up in bed after intercourse and cough to expel the semen, and that if the husband took small doses of arsenic it would encourage impotence, when in reality he frequently died. Allbutt practically suggested that couples practice the use of 'safe' periods, douching after sex and the 'French letter'. For saying these things publicly, he was roundly censured by his colleagues. The General Medical Council met in secret and, after agreeing that there was every possibility his book might be seen by the 'unmarried', banned the volume and struck Allbutt off its Register, ruining him.

Increasingly literate and litigious patients were regarded with increased suspicion and, following a celebrated lawsuit in which a doctor was accused of having murdered a patient who might have been a former mistress, as well as other incidents in which doctors were accused of sexually abusing their patients, the first Medical Defence Union was formed in Britain. For an annual premium, doctors were insured for legal defence in the event of their being sued. Across the Atlantic, such organizations came later, and until then doctors insured themselves through normal insurance companies.

Henceforth, bristling with legal defence bodies, 'beneficent' medicine continued as the norm up to the 1950s in Britain. Those who took action against a doctor on any grounds – and, as people became more medically aware, they began to perceive the mistakes to which they were subjected – were regarded as an infernal nuisance. 'Members of the public will initiate proceedings against doctors on any pretext whatsoever,' wrote a respected physician as late as 1954. Plaintiffs were regarded as deluded, obstinate and stupid, and their allegations as worthless. The solicitors of the medical defence unions found that a ferocious letter usually terrified the often timorous and uncertain victims of incompetence into a state of crushed submission. Of the first 383 defence cases undertaken by the Medical Defence Union, only three produced results unfavourable to it, a fact of which it was eminently proud.

Since the Second World War, the principle of 'informed consent' has given patients concrete rights to necessary information concerning their treatment. The right to informed consent, particularly in America, has allowed patients to question the actions of their doctors, and has given them legal grounds to sue where they would previously have remained silent. Increasingly, doctors and patients have become polarized, and mutually suspicious of each others' behaviour. The silence of 'therapeutic beneficence' has become more a means by which the doctor protects himself from a risk of legal action if he mis-diagnoses or mistreats than a paternalist course of action taken for the benefit of the patient.

In addition, the last century has brought such rapid techno-logical advances in medicine, and such a degree of specializa-tion, that doctors are alienated from patients by the very com-plexity of the chemicals and machinery with which they treat them. Once they spoke in Latin in front of their patients, or were simply silent. Now, if they were to try to explain the mechanics of the medical process, it is unlikely they could make themselves understood. The veritable arsenal of drugs, machinery, and techniques employed in treatment has provided endless opportunities for things to go wrong, and doctors are often uncertain as to whether they are electricians or physi-cians. A famous 1983 Harvard University study found that one mortality in ten reviewed in the research would have been pre-vented if the doctors had simply used their eyes and brains instead of trusting to their plugged-in devices. One American commentator has said that medical malpractice has changed from 'an ethical problem into a technical one'.

Medical litigation

Medical litigation has escalated wildly in America over the last twenty years, and awards to patients have risen to astronomical heights. In 1976, there were four awards of $1 million or more. Five years later, there were forty-five, and over the same period the average settlement rose to $840,396. A quarter of Florida's obstetricians had stopped practicing their speciality because of the danger of litigation; American juries were liable to award particularly large sums in the case of infants. One baby girl was awarded $29.2 million after being made deaf and blind by meningitis.

The size and frequency of damages awards means that malpractice insurance for doctors and surgeons has rocketed in cost. By 1975, premiums were increasing three times a year. In 1976, surgeons found them increased tenfold. The three highest premium areas are those where the biggest payouts customarily occur – California, New York, and Florida, which in turn contain the highest percentage of doctors, something of a bonus to the insurance companies. By 1985, a Long Island obstetrician was paying $82,500 a year in malpractice insurance, and a neurosurgeon in the same area was paying $101,000 annually. However, the hike in premiums was not wholly justified by the massive medico-legal payouts; of the $300 million that ended up in the pockets of the insurance companies in 1970, only 20 per cent was actually paid out to the public. Even fifteen years later, the pattern had changed little, and many doctors claimed that the insurance companies had exaggerated the stories of outrageous claims in order to milk the medical profession. Many malpractice claims are settled before they get to court, because it is cheaper for the companies, a source of dismay to doctors who may have cumulatively paid a million dollars in insurance premiums and want to fight accusations made against them.

Studies of the extent of medical malpractice failed to reach any conclusion, or to lay the blame for the epidemic anywhere in particular, but from the doctor's point of view a number of factors contributed to the legal mayhem.

Firstly, America is the most litigious nation on earth, where people are acutely aware of their individual rights, and where suing your neighbour is as much a part of life as baseball. It has been said that under the American Constitution the average citizen who is angered at his medical treatment may either reach for his gun or file a suit. There are few formal complaints procedures in America, whereas in England people can complain through a number of official bodies which take the momentum out of the patients' onslaught and prevent them reaching the stage of suing. The practice of 'contingency suing' – the 'poor man's door to justice', in which a lawyer will undertake a case free of charge and send in a claim for up to 40 per cent of the award if he wins – is claimed to be part of this problem, as are ambitious and greedy lawyers – 'ambulance chasers and accident watchers' – who prowl hospitals soliciting for clients; 'Support a lawyer – send your son to medical school,' is a popular American saying. Some also blame the free legal education services supplied to the population of some states who are subsequently attracted to sue after reading about the size of awards. Legal fees are also vast in America, which makes litigation an inherently expensive process.

Secondly, there is no public health service as such for Americans. Medicare and Medicaid provide last-ditch options for the old and the poor. Being sick is expensive, and even a couple of additional weeks in hospital for a patient due to a negligent act by a doctor is liable to cost a small fortune.

Thirdly, because there is no health service, the immediate point of treatment for some fifty million poor Americans is the emergency room, where they can only go in desperation. Here they arrive, needing acute care from pressured staff, and, in this difficult and often violent atmosphere, mistakes, or what appear to the patients to be mistakes, are more likely to occur.

The fourth reason that doctors gave for the epidemic was simple adverse publicity, giving rise to copycat claims.

Finally, the public have been led to expect miracles from medicine, and are bitterly disappointed by failure. There is some truth in this point; but also, it has traditionally suited both parties to place the doctor on a pedestal. In modern times the development of medicine into a huge and lucrative business has necessitated an endless supply of good publicity.

But the otherwise inconclusive federal investigations into malpractice did not reveal that the rise in suits was due to a preponderance of wicked lawyers, nor that all the claims were unjustified, nor that the practice of contingency suing was spawning irresponsible claims. On the contrary, they found that the majority of claims were entirely justified, and that the average award was relatively small. Furthermore, the majority of claims arose from incidents which took place in hospitals – where most American medicine is practiced – and were the consequence of avoidable accidents of technology and training. In effect, they were saying that patients had good reason to distrust their doctors, an assertion which is lent weight by the many American studies into the causes of 'iatrogenic illness' (medically induced disease).

The problem of misdiagnosis

Diagnosis should be the foundation of medicine. But, of the top five reasons why Americans sue their doctors, the number one reason is failure to diagnose cancer, number three is failure to diagnose fractures or dislocations, and number four is failure to diagnose a pregnancy-related problem.

A study of American hospitals found that doctors made errors in diagnosis in between 13.1 per cent, and 15.6 per cent of cases. Errors arose for a multitude of apparently petty reasons: from defective equipment, little or bad contact with the patient, a haphazard routine, simple misinterpretation of the signs of sickness, and failure to know what they meant – and, of course, the doctors' favourite, bad handwriting, cited in a study by Davis and Cohen as the most frequent cause of medication error. Some 58 per cent of information on hospital charts and some 80 per cent of doctors' signatures are all illegible. Verbal orders, issued at speed without clear enunciation, are also potentially lethal, because there are many similar-sounding drugs. At one Kentucky hospital the doctor ordered 0.8 milligrams of morphine sulphate for a seventeen-month-old girl, but the nurse thought he said 0.8 millilitres – cubic centimetres – of the drug, which, injected into the child, was liable to prove fatal; it was, and did.

In 1985, a study by the University of Washington's Department of Family Medicine attempted to find out how well physicians knew the risks involved in ten surgical and 'invasive' diagnostic procedures. In the survey of 128 doctors, only 27 per cent of responses were correct. Of the remainder, 26 per cent underestimated the dangers, and 21 per cent admitted no knowledge whatsoever as to the dangers involved.

Psychiatric misdiagnosis is common. An American doctor, Robert S. Hoffman, blames the process on a chain of irreversible and tragic events, whereby 'a primary physician applies a preliminary diagnosis of mental disorder which is decisive in determining the patient's subsequent course'. Once the stigma of psychiatric disorder is applied to an individual it can be impossible to remove it. Of 215 psychiatric patients in institutions in America, tests revealed that 41 per cent should probably not have been referred in the first place, and that of those with a diagnosis of 'untreatable dementia', 63 per cent had wholly treatable conditions. At a Manhattan psychiatric centre, 131 patients selected at random were examined, and it was concluded that up to 75 per cent of them had been misdiagnosed when first admitted to hospital.

A principal error is to mistake signs of physical illness as emergent psychiatric problems. Instead of looking to practical remedies, which may be connected to lifestyle, emotional problems or some biochemical imbalance, the doctor prefers to lump what he does not understand under the heading of mental illness and thrust the patient into an institution, or put him or her on mind-altering drugs which may have irreversible side-effects. The drugs given to treat schizophrenia – such as Thorazine – may have side-effects such as tremors and spasms which will subsequently obviate attempts to re-examine the patient. Research by the University of Ottowa argued that 43 per cent of psychiatric patients had one or more severe physical disorders, the symptoms of which were mistakenly seen as related to a psychiatric problem, or were indeed caused by the psychiatric drugs, and that in 20 per cent of these cases physical illness alone was the cause of the supposed psychiatric disorder.

Insecurity in diagnosis leads to excessive faith in laboratory testing, which has become a substitute for clinical diagnosis. The average American entering hospital is liable to be faced with at least twenty tests of one sort or another, and has a less than 36 per cent chance of emerging from these as wholly normal, even if he or she is initially in blooming health. It is claimed that excessive testing of perfectly healthy people results in the creation of phantom illnesses, which rapidly grow into real ones the moment patients are subjected to a battery of drugs. Puzzled doctors are prone to what is known as 'serendipitomania', the common habit of ordering all available laboratory tests in the hope of simply falling into a disease. The result will often be a 'cascade' effect, where one test leads to another and another, each of which leads further and further away from the original complaint.

The number of tests used in American hospitals has risen by 10-15 per cent annually. This does not stem solely from insecurity, nor from fear of litigation (cited in one study as the cause of only 1 per cent of testing), but also from curiosity. With so many new diagnostic procedures available in the laboratory, doctors are in effect often testing the tests. Since a patient in a hospital is liable to be seen by up to twenty different physicians, each doctor will want to cover himself by ordering his own preferred set of tests. Because such testing is lucrative, doctors are rarely criticized by their hospitals for over-ordering tests, and research has conclusively shown that doctors in groups which charge separately for each aspect of treatment are likely to order a great many more tests than those organizations which charge a flat fee for treatment: up to a staggering 50 per cent more electrocardiogram tests and X-rays.

Excessive testing is sometimes a product of a bad patient-doctor relationship. Patients who pay considerable sums for private treatment want to feel that something is being done, and the doctor placates them by prescribing superfluous tests, which gives the patient the opportunity to see the scanners, electrocardiographs, and X-ray machines they have paid for. In the case of ultrasound pictures of babies during pregnancy, some 30 per cent are probably unnecessary; the *New York*

Times concluded that it was simply curiosity on the part of parents that drove them to the tests. The ultrasound pictures made a unique addition to the family snapshot album, but had no medical value.

As there is little coherent notion of what a normal, healthy person is, the conclusions drawn from tests are a matter of subjective opinion. In one study published in the medical periodical *The Lancet*, 197 out of 200 patients were cured of their illnesses by simply reconducting the 'infallible' laboratory tests.

Many physicians have found that a quick way to increase their income is to start their own home-grown testing businesses in their backyards. An 'in-house' lab such as this is claimed by doctors to provide test results more quickly than would be the case if one had to mail the specimens off to hospital, or to an independent laboratory; such arrangements are also infinitely cheaper. An investigation conducted on such laboratories in California showed that over 40 per cent of the people employed in them had no formal education or training in performing laboratory analysis, and that up to 80 per cent of their results were substantially less accurate than results from independent labs. There are up to 100,000 of such incompetent laboratories in America.

Once the patient has been classified as suffering from some sickness and been admitted to a hospital for treatment, the hazards begin to pile up. Not the least of these is the possibility of medication error. According to a classic study by Davis and Cohen, medication error in a typical American hospital not using a standard unit dose system of drug distribution is around 12 per cent. In a hospital with 300 patients, where each patient receives an average of ten doses of various drugs daily (the average adult is pumped full of around thirteen different drugs in various combinations) this comes to 131,400 medication errors annually, or 360 a day.

There are many opportunities for error. Patients get the wrong drug or the wrong dosage, or no drug when they should have had a drug, or a number of drugs when they should have had none whatsoever; they get two drugs together which combine disastrously, or they get somebody else's drugs; they get the wrong – or even the right – drug by the wrong method, injected into the wrong place or stuffed into the wrong orifice. The side-effects are not correctly monitored, or the drugs are contaminated or old, or the syringes or catheter by which the drugs are administered are reused and are dirty. Besides getting sick, the patients may react psychologically to the drugs, or become addicted, or they may give birth to mutilated children. 'Polypharmacy' – the multiple application of multiples of combined drugs – can cause such inexplicable and confusing side-effects that the original symptoms of sickness become indiscernible beneath the web of iatrogenic sickness, which is then treated by the further application of yet more drugs, and in stronger doses.

Side-effects include acute gastrointestinal problems, muscle disorders, headaches, emotional and psychic disorders, heart trouble, hepatitis (and a myriad other disorders of the liver, through which the chemicals pass), cataracts and lupus (a tuberculosis of the skin which is produced by over forty drugs).

Principal among the causes of polypharmacy are the physician's lack of knowledge of the effects of what he is prescribing, his consequent failure to set 'therapeutic objectives' (that is, a point at which treatment will be said to be complete) and his natural reluctance to believe that the treatment he has prescribed is doing any harm.

In addition, many drugs are simply prescribed on a prophylactic basis; nothing appears to be wrong, but, just in case, a course of antibiotics is administered. Or the doctor is baffled by what he sees, and after discovering that the patient has once suffered from a particular infection, he prescribes antibiotics in case the previous illness recurs. Research shows that at least 50 per cent of prescribed prophylactic antibiotics were given when there was no infection, or when a less expensive drug would have done, and that the dose was far too great or the treatment extended for no good reason. Money may be an incentive; outside the hospital, a doctor who issues his own prescriptions may be making $40,000 per year in the process.

The over-use of 'broad-spectrum' prophylactic antibiotics is not only costly, and dangerous, but is an act of scientific suicide; it provides the microbes with endless opportunities to become drug-resistant, to develop increased sophistication, and to render the precious 'magic bullet' of penicillin, and its relations, useless. Some antibiotics are already redundant; others are only any use in vast and expensive doses.

Misdiagnosed, awash with alien chemicals, but convinced they are getting value for money in the morbid theme park of contemporary American medicine, patients who have hitherto survived are shortly to encounter the next challenge to their lives: nosocomial infections. These are hospital-induced infections, conveyed from patient to patient by unwashed hands, bad personal and environmental hygiene, crowded conditions, pleasantly lukewarm, reheated food, and lousy ventilation. About 5-10 per cent of the American hospital population develops a nosocomial infection and around 100,000 people die from nosocomial-related infections each year; it has been said that the genuine figure is about three times this size. Chief among fatal infections is pneumonia, which attacks 0.5-5 per cent of all hospital in-patients. It kills between a fifth and a half of all those it infects and is responsible for up to 15 per cent of all deaths in hospital.

Inadequate hand-washing procedures are a prime spreader of disease. Laboratory researchers who have spent a morning swilling blood and urine around have been seen to stroll out of the lab to lunch without washing their hands. Surgeons put too much faith in the gloves they wear; and machinery is improperly sterilized, particularly intravenous infusion devices, respiratory equipment and dialysis machines. Catheters, particularly urinary ones, are a common source of infection; disposable devices intended to be used only once are cleaned up and employed again by money-conscious hospitals. Thermometers, bedpans, suction tubes and surgical instruments are badly washed. Hepatitis B is fond of dialysis units, salmonella loves hospital food, and legionnaire's disease is happily at home in the water-cooling towers and ventilation systems. By 1985, nosocomial infections were costing Americans around $2.5 billion annually and were one of America's major causes of premature death.

Between 20 and 25 million operations are carried out in America each year. Of these, somewhere between 15 per cent and 25 per cent are said to be unnecessary, and in the case of some operations, such as tonsillectomies and hysterectomies, the unnecessary portion is as high as 80 per cent. This amounts to between 3 million and 6 million unnecessary operations per annum. Given that surgery generally has a mortality rate of around 1.33 per cent, it has been claimed that there are up to 80,000 deaths per annum from unnecessary surgery. If these figures are realistic, more people die each year from unnecessary surgery than died in Korea and Vietnam. There is also the cost; in 1974, a US Senate investigation into this phenomenon reported that doctors performed nearly two and a half million unnecessary operations each year, costing nearly $4 billion.

The most common unnecessary operations are tonsillectomies, Caesarean sections, and hysterectomies, which make the most frequent victims women. It has been noted that whereas predominantly male surgeons baulk at the thought of whipping off a testicle, they have less empathy with women and few qualms about excising an ovary. Caesarean section is now regarded as a normal option for an obstetrician when birth is potentially problematic; it is far easier to operate than risk a malpractice suit should you prove unlucky with the forceps.

The need to make money fast to pay off debts accumulated throughout time at medical school has often been cited as a reason for the speed with which American surgeons reach for the knife. As the number of surgeons plying their trade has increased, so has the number of operations performed. During the period when the post-war population of America rose by 43 per cent, the number of operations rose by 122 per cent, there was an increased number of young surgeons all competing in the marketplace. The number of surgeons expands at over twice the rate of the general population.

There are minor operations which can be urged upon the patient by the acquisitive surgeon: the removal of healthy tonsils; cataract lens implants; cosmetic surgery; and circumcision. The last should not be necessary other than for religious reasons; yet 1.5 million circumcisions are performed on newborn males every year in America, on 80 per cent of male infants. It can be hazardous, as in the case of two infants in an Atlanta hospital in 1985. Both were badly burned by the cauterizing needles used in circumcision, one of them so mutilated that his penis was destroyed. A sex change operation was subsequently performed and the child is currently being raised as a female, incapable of reproduction and in need of lifelong hormonal therapy.

Heart bypass and 'balloon' surgery is a current favourite, though in many cases it is not as effective as putting the patient on a low-fat diet, throwing out their cigarettes and compelling them to take exercise.

The seductive perils of technology were seen far back, before the turn of the century. Noting the arrival of the microscope, the laryngoscope, the spectroscope, the medical uses of electricity, and the humble thermometer, the *British Medical Journal* commented that these were but 'ingenious and beautiful toys ... medicine is fast wandering away from the mission to cure a disease and becoming engrossed by phenomena, forgetting the patient while the disease is studied.'

It is argued that the preference for studying disease and death may be traced back further than the thermometer, to the time in the eighteenth century when pathological anatomy – dissection and examination of the dead and the study of the effects of death and disease – took the medical gaze away from contemplating the contradictions of the living. Doctors who had struggled for hundreds of years to classify sickness and to know its origins found that by opening up a few corpses, they could at last 'see' the disease. The living then became the bearers of disease, potentially sick rather than inherently alive. As Kant said, 'Doctors think they are doing you a favour when they label something you have as a disease.' Since the process of dissection became the foundation of medical education, living patients have come to be viewed in a mechanistic fashion:

nothing can be finally known about them until they have been scanned, X-rayed, and mechanically probed, or until they lie on the autopsy slab.

The first patient encounter American medical students have is with a corpse, which is in many ways the ideal patient, one who will not answer back and in the presence of whom one maintains emotional distance; communication skills are not easily learned from corpses. Unconscious females are used for gynaecology education. The training, as the American Cynthia Carver has written, 'is disease orientated, with life-threatening or rare conditions receiving the most attention, and the acquisition of skill in doing procedures ... and using diagnostic machines ... being prized ... The promotion of health and the prevention of disease are almost entirely neglected.'

The living, conscious patient is a problematic organism, but the student has a diminishing interest in the patient as human, and less knowledge of the web of emotional, familial, and social forces that precipitate sickness; the living patients student doctors do encounter are likely to be in the emergency room of a hospital, people who need acute care. The fascination with studying, classifying and isolating sickness rather than pursuing health, and a preoccupation with machinery, are twin aspects of the current crisis in medical training.

It has been customary to tackle those contradictions of contemporary medicine in a curative fashion: with regulation, money, the expulsion of malefactors, and the demand for better hospitals with better-trained staff. But recently, some have begun to question the very basis of the medical culture that creates the problem.

Modern medicine has, as one commentator has put it, converted us from a 'society of mortality into one of morbidity'.

Afraid of death, we rigorously pursue health; but medicine has perversely mutated into an industry which even creates its own diseases. In this scheme, it is argued, doctors have unconsciously become the salespeople of products and techniques, and the aloofness and authority with which their training invests them make it difficult for them to acknowledge the fundamental failures of the profession.

Should medicine and medical training, worldwide, and not only in America, not concern themselves more with preventative medicine than with the treatment of disease alone? For, at the moment, the doctor is in danger of being reduced to a sales outlet in a 'culture of sickness' where blunders proliferate.

Chapter Five

Drugs worse than diseases

Dangerous blisters

Some of the worst medical blunders, particularly in this century, have been caused by unknown side-effects from new drugs. Throughout the history of medicine drugs seem to have caused almost as much harm as good. The practice of blistering as a medical treatment was once common. Blisters were usually raised by means of plasters smeared with a preparation of Spanish fly, or cantharides, a highly irritating substance. Some doctors, while acknowledging the merits of blistering, were, however, careful to make certain reservations.

Here is an extract from the book *Observations on Maniacal Disorders* by William Pargeter MD, published in 1792; after dilating on the value of blistering, properly applied in selected cases of mental disease, Pargeter warns: 'But in those species of the disorder named *nymphomania* or *metromania et satyriasis*, the use of blisters must be most strictly prohibited; and indeed in every case of madness where there is a disposition to salacity, which is a very common concomitant symptom, this ought to be cautiously and seriously attended to... Indeed, in all cases, blistering plasters, before they are applied, should be either sprinkled with camphor, or a fine piece of muslin should be interposed between them and the skin, by which means *stranguria* (painful and difficult urination), or what is infinitely more disagreeable, *priapismus* (persistent erection), will most generally be prevented. Two fatal instances of the excessive use of cantharides producing *satyriasis* (a compulsive desire to have sexual intercourse with as many women as possible) are recorded by Cabrolius Obs. Anat, 17, and others in the *Ephemerides Germanicae Curiosae Decad 1.*'

Pargeter has a point. Cantharides has, from time immemorial, been widely regarded as an effective aphrodisiac. The dried and powdered body of the European beetle, *Cantharis vesicatoria* contains the powerfully irritating, blistering and toxic substance cantharidin which is readily absorbed through the skin or mucous membranes. The chemical name for pure crystalline cantharidin (hexahydro-3a,7a-dimethyl-4,7-epoxy-isobenzofuran-1,3-dione) is about as fearful as its effects on the body.

Once absorbed, and this readily occurs through the skin, the drug produces widespread damage to any tissue with which it comes in contact. It is then excreted in the urine and as it does so it causes an acute inflammation of the whole urinary tract, including a form of nephritis that can prove fatal. A conspicuous feature of this is inflammation of the urethra – the tube along which urine is passed from the bladder. Anyone suffering from such a urethritis would certainly have his or her attention drawn constantly to the genitalia. Whether this would have the effect of promoting sexual arousal (presumably the basis of this substance's reputation as an aphrodisiac) is another matter entirely.

There is a report in the literature about the office manager of a firm of wholesale chemical manufacturers who was so unwise as to make up a confection of cantharides in coconut ice which he fed to two young office girls. The outcome – an indictment for manslaughter and a sentence of five years' imprisonment, was somewhat less pleasant than he had presumably hoped for. Both girls had died after suffering terrible agonies.

Many patients must, in the past, have suffered grievously from the medical use of cantharides – a substance for the use of which there can be no possible medical justification. The medical value of blistering, by whatever means, is negligible.

Freud and the cocaine blunder

The dream of a 'universal panacea' has never ceased to haunt mankind, and doctors – who ought to know better – are by no means immune to belief in this chimera. Unfortunately, the only drugs that have achieved any plausibility as cure-alls have been those with powerful actions. Equally unfortunately, powerful drugs – such as opium and cocaine – always have powerful disadvantages, as those who have been persuaded to use them have discovered to their cost.

For thousands of years, the leaves of the coca plants *Erythroxylon coca* and *E. truxiuense* – indigenous to the Andes in South America, especially Peru and Bolivia – have been chewed by the local inhabitants to relieve hunger and provide energy and strength. Sigmund Freud's interest in cocaine was aroused by reports on its use to invigorate German Army troops during manoeuvres. Freud read about these experiments in *Deutsche Medizinische Wochenschrift* and decided to try the drug on patients with heart disease and with 'nervous exhaustion' following withdrawal from morphine.

But, quite properly, he decided first to try it on himself, especially when he was tired, depressed and bothered by stomach cramps. In the true spirit of scientific enquiry, he began to take small doses of pure cocaine. Because he was using the pure substance rather than chewing the leaves it was possible for him to get a reasonably accurate idea of the appropriate dosage needed. To his delight, all his symptoms were relieved.

Experiments on colleagues

The results so pleased and impressed him that he began to administer cocaine to friends, colleagues and patients. One of these was the pathologist von Fleischel-Marxow, a twenty-five-year-old research worker who had had to have his right thumb amputated following a severe infection. The cut nerves of the thumb caused him constant severe pain. In his anxiety to get on with his work he had started taking morphine to relieve the pain and he had become thoroughly addicted to it. In May 1883 Freud started to treat Fleischel-Marxow with cocaine. Freud might have guessed that this would be futile, as there was no reason to suppose that cocaine could deal with the real cause of the symptom – the irritation of the cut nerves. Treating symptoms rather than causes is bad medicine. Predictably, the only effect was to substitute cocaine addiction for morphine addiction.

Undaunted, Freud continued with his research into the drug. He developed a simple but clever device he called a dynamometer, that could be used to measure the power of the grip and another, even more ingenious, gadget to measure reaction time. These he used to assess the effects of cocaine on himself. In a letter to his fiancée Martha Bernays in 1884 he wrote: 'Woe to you, my Princess, when I come. I will kiss you

quite red and feed you till you are plump. And if you are forward, you shall see who is the stronger, a gentle little girl who
doesn't eat enough or a big wild man who has cocaine in his
body. In my last severe depression I took coca again and a
small dose lifted me to the heights in a wonderful fashion. I am
busy collecting the literature for a song of praise to this wonderful substance.' Freud was very hard up at the time and had
been borrowing money heavily from more prosperous colleagues. It occurred to him that here was a possible way of
achieving not only medical fame, but financial independence.

Publications
In his paper *'Über Coca'* published the same year in
Centralblatt Fur die Gesamte Therapie he gave an account of
the use of the leaves of the coca plant by South American
Indians and described its effects on animals and humans. His
conclusion was that the greatest value of the drug was in temporarily strengthening the body. He also recommended it as a
means of relieving indigestion after dietary indiscretion and in
the treatment of anaemia, asthma and addiction to alcohol and
morphine. Possibly because of his long separation from his
fiancée, he was convinced that the drug was an aphrodisiac.
Having noticed the numbing effect of the drug on the mouth he
realized that this loss of sensation could have applications in
surgery, and in this paper he referred briefly to the anaesthetic
properties of the drug. He was later to regret that he had
neglected this aspect and, instead, had emphasized the value of
the general effect.

At that time, the range of operations that could be performed
on the eye was very limited. For various reasons, the type of
general anaesthesia available then was unsuitable and was

liable to cause complications that could threaten vision. It seemed to Freud likely that cocaine could produce adequate anaesthesia without causing these dangers. At this juncture, unfortunately, he had not seen Martha for a year and had arranged to visit her in Wandsbek. So, instead of continuing with planned work on the use of cocaine as an aid to ophthalmic surgery, he briefed a colleague Carl Koller about the idea and went off to see his girlfriend.

Cocaine eyedrops

In his absence, Koller and his assistant Joseph Gaertner made up some eyedrops consisting of a solution of cocaine. After trying it out on some animals, they instilled it into each other's eyes. To their astonishment they found that they could touch the corneas of their eyes without experiencing any sensation whatsoever. They were even able to indent the corneas slightly with no feeling of touch. Clearly this was a major advance that would enable eye surgeons to work without difficulty. Koller sent a paper to an ophthalmological convention in Heidelberg announcing how easily the cornea could be completely anaesthetized for surgery. Within weeks the news had spread around Europe, the drug came into routine use, and Koller was famous. The soft drink Coca-cola had been originated by a Atlanta pharmacist in 1886 and was rapidly becoming popular. Inevitably, Koller became known as 'Coca Koller'.

Soon it became clear that cocaine was an excellent local anaesthetic and that it could be used far more widely than only on the eye. Two American surgeons, Richard J. Hall and William S. Halstead, working at the John's Hopkins Medical School in Baltimore were especially active in developing the use of the drug, by injection, for general surgery. In order to establish the required dosage and the best methods of injection they conducted many experiments on each other. Eventually they came to perform thousands of major operations under injections of cocaine anaesthesia. By that time, however, both of them were hopelessly addicted to the drug. Halstead turned to morphine in an attempt to kick the cocaine habit and did so at the cost of morphine addiction. He remained addicted to morphine for the rest of his life – a fact that his colleagues kept secret from the general public. In spite of this Halstead had a distinguished career and made some other notable advances in surgery. He invented rubber operating gloves and developed an effective, if mutilating, operation for breast cancer – the radical mastectomy.

Freud was thus denied credit for the one really valuable application of the drug – its use as a local anaesthetic. Ironically, the other uses he suggested came, in the end, to be seen, by himself as well as others, to be as undesirable as they were misguided. For his advocacy of cocaine as a stimulant, Freud was mercilessly attacked by more cautious colleagues and came bitterly to regret his haste. After about 1886 he no longer took cocaine, or advocated its use as a general stimulant.

The blind baby blunder

If there is one literally vital requirement for survival, it is oxygen. A person can live for weeks without food and for days without water, but only for a few short minutes without oxygen.

Premature babies are small babies. What matters is not how

long they have been developing in the womb, but how far that development has proceeded. Underdevelopment affects everything in the body including the lungs, and it also affects the production of a wetting agent – a surfactant – that helps the originally solid lungs to expand into their normal spongy state so that air can get into them.

The first concern, therefore, in the care of premature babies, is to ensure that they get enough oxygen. This is one reason why they are almost always nursed in incubators where the concentration of oxygen in the air they are breathing can be kept high. Ordinary atmospheric air contains about 20 per cent of oxygen. Most of the rest is inert nitrogen. Oxygen therapy consists in giving air containing higher than 20 per cent oxygen. In theory, one could give up to 100 per cent oxygen.

The practice of giving high oxygen concentrations to premature babies began around 1940 and it was common to give these babies anything up to 70 per cent of oxygen in the air they breathed. In 1941 a baby in Boston, Massachusetts was found to be blind. This little baby girl had been premature but had done well and was now thriving. Examination showed, however, that immediately behind the internal lens of each eye was a greyish-white mass of fibrous tissue containing numerous tiny blood vessels. These masses were dense enough to preclude any image being formed on the baby's retinas so the child was unable to see.

Soon after this, another Boston baby, one of a pair of premature twins, was found to have the same condition. This child's twin sister had been even smaller at birth and had died after six hours from inability to breathe adequately. This child was examined by an eye specialist, Dr Theodore Terry, and was confirmed as being blind. Dr Terry was told about the earlier case and his professional interest was aroused. By 1945 he had seen no fewer than 117 cases and had published a report on the condition. In every single case the condition had occurred in babies who had been premature. Because the problem lay behind the lens it was called retrolental (*retro-* means 'behind' and *lentis* means 'a lens'). And because there was growth or spread of fibrous tissue it was called fibroplasia (*plasia* simply means 'growth', 'development' or 'change').

The doctors were deeply puzzled. Was retrolental fibroplasia a new disease of premature babies? A study of previous records of such babies showed that it was practically unknown. In 1946 a case occurred in Britain and soon afterwards cases began to crop up all over Europe, in Canada, South Africa, Israel and Australia. By 1953 it was estimated that 50 per cent of all cases of blindness in children under seven was caused by retrolental fibroplasia. After the National Health Service was instituted in England, cases of retrolental fibroplasia became common.

First conclusions

By now the doctors had concluded that this distressing condition was simply a consequence of prematurity. It was assumed that, with improving methods of caring for premature babies, more and more were surviving to show the disorder. It also became apparent that the lower the birth weight, the greater was the likelihood of developing blindness from retrolental fibroplasia. Strangely, not all very small premature babies developed the condition. And there were certain premature baby units that had never had a single case. Even more mysterious was the fact that the largest numbers of cases were occurring in the baby units that were best endowed and had the finest equipment and the most highly qualified staff. To the surprise of everyone, it was found that some of the poorest units, working on minimal endowment and watching every penny, had no cases at all.

One of the theories put forward to account for the condition was that the eyes of very premature babies were being damaged from lack of oxygen. It seemed logical, therefore, to step up even further the concentration of oxygen in the atmosphere breathed by these babies. In spite of this, the condition became more and more common. Careful studies of these babies now showed that more premature babies developed the condition than had been thought but that many of these with early retrolental fibroplasia showed a regression of the condition and a full recovery. Indeed, it soon became apparent that about 85 per cent of those with the early condition recovered. In only 15 per cent did the condition progress to its full extent and cause blindness. It was also discovered that in severe cases the mass behind the lens was complicated by other eye changes including massive retinal detachment. This left a hopeless situation with no possible prospects of later treatment. By 1950, at least 2,500 babies were being blinded each year from retrolental fibroplasia. All these cases were occurring in high tech hospitals. There was a blunder somewhere.

Steps forward

In 1951 there was an important step forward. It was found that premature babies given 40 per cent oxygen were much less likely to develop retrolental fibroplasia than babies given 60 or 70 per cent oxygen. This was a surprise and ran counter to medical opinion, but the facts were beyond dispute. In one trial, alternate premature babies were given the lower percentage and the others the higher. There was no doubt about it; the babies on low oxygen developed fibroplasia far less often than those on high oxygen.

A researcher at the Institute of Ophthalmology in London, Norman Ashton, now came up with a remarkable theory. Tissues that are short of oxygen or are inadequately nourished try to compensate for these deficiencies by budding out fronds of new blood vessels. This is a normal process and these new vessels are relatively effective in supplying the extra blood and improving the local nutrition. Under normal circumstances these extra vessels are beneficial. When no longer needed they disappear or develop into normal larger vessels. Premature babies' retinas are seriously short of nutrition so considerable new vessel growth occurs. If, however, extra oxygen is given, these new vessels close down as do many of the normal blood vessels needed to keep the retina healthy and working normally. So long as the high level of extra oxygen is supplied, the normal profusion of blood vessels is unnecessary. The real trouble starts, however, when the high oxygen is turned off and the baby has to try to manage on normal atmospheric levels. At this point, because many of the normal retinal blood vessels have been closed off and obliterated, the retinas are seriously short of blood. Immediately, they respond by a massive growth of abnormal and very thin-walled new blood vessels that extend from the edge of the retina into the jelly of the eye. These abnormal new vessels bleed easily and soon the region behind the lens is filled with a network of small vessels and fibrous tissue.

Ashton's ideas were backed up by careful experimental work and were reported in *The British Journal of Ophthalmology* and elsewhere. They are now recognized as having wide implications in the understanding of how tissues are nourished.

Once the cause of retrolental fibroplasia was understood and the levels of oxygen cut down to a minimum, the epidemic of blind babies came to an abrupt end. Suddenly, as if by magic, the figures dropped almost to zero. In New York this condition caused 168 cases of blindness in 1952 and 167 in 1953. In 1955, the first full year in which the new low-oxygen policy was universally implemented, just three babies were blinded from this cause.

The drugging of Adolf Hitler

For almost a decade, the fate of millions depended on the whim of Adolf Hitler. There is excellent reason to believe that this man was addicted to amphetamine, administered by his personal physician Theodor Morell. From late 1941 or early 1942 Hitler was visited by Morell almost every morning and was given an intravenous injection before getting out of bed. Almost instantaneously, Hitler felt alert and active and ready for the day's work. About the middle of 1943, Hitler started to have injections at other times of the day. All his close associates were impressed by the effects of Morell's injections. These effects lasted for several hours. Hitler became alert, very talkative, cheerful and physically active and was able to stay awake long into the night. Although Morell claimed that these injections were of vitamins, no vitamin could account for these clearly recorded and persistent effects, even in a highly suggestible person. The duration of the effect was such as to eliminate cocaine as a possibility.

Amphetamine, under the trade name of Pervitin, was widely

available in Germany from about 1937 and it is known that Hitler was aware of its properties from about that time. The drug was actually issued to military units (on both sides) as a stimulant to be used when the military situation required that the soldiers should go without sleep for long periods. A German Panzer veteran reports that he and his fellow soldiers ate amphetamine 'like sweets' when they had to fight all night.

Hitler's addictions
The medical evidence strongly suggests that Hitler suffered from amphetamine toxicity, at least from the late summer of 1942. His sudden changes of mood, from euphoria to depression, are characteristic. He showed personality changes typical of those caused by persistent amphetamine overdose – withdrawal, suspicion, violent rages and paranoia. One of his most characteristic gestures was persistently to bite the skin around the nail of either thumb and of the first two fingers of each hand. This habit, said to be a feature of amphetamine toxicity, persisted to the end of his life. Although it led to chronic inflammation and tenderness, he was, apparently, unable to stop. Neither the pain nor his preoccupation with his image were strong enough to check the habit.

Hitler's attitude to personal responsibility, once strong, changed and he began to blame his subordinates for the military reverses that were the results of his own errors of judgement. Amphetamine can also increase aggressiveness and promote a tendency to take risks. The lack of judgement that led to the Russian campaign, the disaster of the battle of Stalingrad and subsequent events can all be attributed to the effects of this drug. As the war situation worsened he began to have intravenous injections of amphetamine to counter bad news and to take barbiturates to let him sleep.

Hitler has been widely described as having been insane and most psychiatric diagnoses have been applied to him. He was, however, forty-nine years old before any unequivocal mental disorder appeared. This fact alone is sufficient virtually to eliminate a diagnosis of psychotic or psychoneurotic illness. The only plausible explanation is that there was an external cause for these manifestations; and all the evidence suggests that this cause was amphetamine.

The conduct of war has commonly been affected by the health of military and political leaders. There seems little doubt that as a result of poor health, Franklin D. Roosevelt was no match for the wily and unscrupulous Joseph Stalin at the vital Yalta conference in February, 1945, at which the Communist domination of post-war eastern Europe was determined. Roosevelt was suffering from congestive heart failure – the illness from which he died two months later, and everyone was shocked by his appearance. There is evidence that because of his illness he was barely briefed for the conference and had made little preparation. Further, instead of giving Churchill the support and backing he needed, he seemed sometimes almost to side with Stalin against Churchill.

The seventy-one-year-old Churchill, too, was in much reduced condition. As his doctor, Lord Moran, records, his powers were waning seriously at the time of Yalta and of the Potsdam Conference later the same year. He had become increasingly deaf and may not always have followed the interpreter. Just over four years later, on 24 August 1949, Churchill suffered a minor stroke. This was followed by the more serious strokes from which he died.

Bad news about beta blockers

The beta blockers are an important group of drugs widely prescribed to counter some of the actions of adrenaline. By block-
ing these adrenaline actions, they slow down an over-rapid
heart, reduce blood pressure, relieve angina, calm panic, reduce
anxiety and control the symptoms of migraine.

The first beta-blocking drug, propranolol, was produced in
1958 by the distinguished Scottish drug scientist James Whyte
Black (1924–) working at Imperial Chemical Industries. In
1948, the American pharmacologist Raymond Ahlquist had
suggested that adrenaline acted on two kinds of hormone
receptors, the alpha receptors and the beta receptors. These had
different effects. Adrenaline entering the beta receptors on the
heart muscle cells caused the heart to speed up and the heart
muscle to contract more strongly. Black was familiar with this
idea and accepted it. He decided to see whether it would be
possible to produce a drug that was similar to adrenaline in that
it would attach itself to the beta receptors but would not cause
them to trigger off their normal effects. If these receptors could
be occupied by the drug molecules, adrenaline would not be
able to act.

Black was brilliantly successful in showing that this could be
done and in producing a whole new class of valuable drugs –
the beta blockers. These revolutionized the treatment of high
blood pressure and other conditions. Not content with this success, Black went on to develop the histamine-blocking drug
cimetidine (Tagamet), used to reduce stomach acid, and thus
founded another new dynasty of drugs of which the best known
is the record-breaking ranitidine (Zantac). For these successes
Black was knighted in 1981, and in 1988 was awarded the

Nobel Prize for physiology or medicine.

Following the remarkable success of the early beta blockers, pharmaceutical chemists got busy developing new drugs of the same class. Once the basic chemical structure of beta blockers was known it was a fairly routine matter to produce further types that might be even more efficient or safer. This was in the post-thalidomide period and drug manufacturers were acutely sensitive to the possibility of dangerous side effects. These new beta-blocker drugs were therefore subjected to the most careful scrutiny and were very thoroughly tested for safety. In 1970 a new beta-blocker drug practolol was put on the market and proved highly successful. Like many other powerful drugs, it had minor side effects such as occasional skin rashes. After four years of use, it was being extensively prescribed and had been taken successfully by at least 50,000 patients.

Other applications

In 1974 an eye specialist who was particularly interested in external eye diseases noticed that an unusual new kind of syndrome seemed to have appeared. This was a condition that caused patients to complain of dryness of the eyes, and it featured familiar changes in the transparent membrane, the conjunctiva, that covers the white of the eye and the inside of the eyelids. The odd thing about these cases was that instead of affecting the exposed parts of the conjunctiva, it seemed to be largely limited to those parts that were protected by the lids. Ophthalmologists had long been familiar with environmentally-induced changes in the exposed conjunctiva but this was something new. In some cases, the damage to the membrane was so severe that it lost its nonstick properties and adhesions developed between layers that were supposed to slide smoothly over each other. In a few cases, the effect was so severe that blindness resulted.

The ophthalmologist's investigations were thorough and included enquiries into medical treatment the affected people might be having. All of them were taking practolol. When the news got about, doctors prescribing this drug began to look for other signs of trouble in their patients and this was soon reported. Covering the organs inside the abdomen is a thin membrane very similar in structure to the conjunctiva of the eyes. This is called the peritoneum. Unfortunately, a few patients taking practolol were found to have developed an inflammatory disorder of the peritoneum similar to what had been found in the conjunctivae of other patients. In these cases, and fortunately there were few, the effect of the inflammation was even more serious and some patients died. Other patients developed inner ear disorders.

The manufacturer quickly acknowledged that these distressing conditions were side effects of practolol and immediately withdrew it from the market. It was apparent that this was a most unlikely and unpredictable complication of the drug and that it affected only a small minority of patients who were susceptible to a particular immune system upset. The firm acknowledged a moral – but not a legal – responsibility to the patients affected and paid compensation.

The thalidomide story

In the autumn of 1961, doctors in West Germany realized that something very strange was happening. An epidemic of extraordinary malformations in babies was occurring. Some of these children had various internal abnormalities but most had the previously rare condition of phocomelia or 'seal limbs', in which the arms and legs were replaced by what looked like short flippers. The long bones of the limbs were absent or greatly shortened and the hands and feet, either virtually normal or rudimentary, were attached close to the body. In 1959, in West Germany, 17 cases had been seen. In 1960, 126. In 1961, 477 cases had occurred. Smaller outbreaks were reported from other countries.

The search for an explanation

No one could suggest a plausible explanation. All kinds of suggestions were made. Virus infections, radioactive fall-out, X-rays, food preservatives, contraceptives were all considered, but none seemed likely to be the cause. The first really convincing evidence that a drug was the cause of these congenital defects came from the Australian obstetrician William McBride. The German paediatrician Widukind Lenz, of Hamburg University, also began to suspect that a drug might be the cause. Pregnant women who had been taking the sedative drug sold as Contergan, Distaval, Softenon, Kevadon, Talimol and under many other names, had no suspicion that it might be dangerous. In Germany it was being bought over the counter in supermarkets. It was thought particularly suitable for women with morning sickness. The drug was produced by the German pharmaceutical firm Grünenthal.

In Britain, the drug Distaval was sold by Distillers Company (Biochemicals) Ltd. and was widely advertised as the safest sedative yet produced, and was prescribed to millions, including many women in early pregnancy. There was so little reason to suspect this drug that these women often failed to mention the fact that they were taking it when completing research questionnaires. One of the main selling points about it had been its safety. When they were directly questioned, however, almost all the women who had had deformed babies were found to have taken Contergan or Distaval or one of the others between the fourth and ninth weeks of pregnancy, when the foetus's limbs were developing. All these drugs were the same. They were thalidomide.

Distillers Company (Biochemicals) Ltd did not have a long-term experience of drug manufacture. Their experience was, of course, in the drink trade and they had broken into pharmaceuticals when, during the war, the government had asked them to help with the production of penicillin. Since this was produced from a mould, their experience in fermentation would be helpful. Distillers Company were not really equipped to develop new drugs for themselves so they were interested in handling a new drug produced elsewhere. It was their extreme misfortune to pick on thalidomide.

Thalidomide banned world-wide
In November 1961 the drug was withdrawn in West Germany and, in December 1961, it was withdrawn in Britain. The American paediatrician Helen Taussig, who was also investigating cases of phocomelia in Britain and Germany, also concluded that thalidomide was the cause. Her advice to the American Food and Drug Administration (FDA), together with the suspicions of an alert FDA executive called Frances Kelsey, resulted in a refusal to license the drug for the USA. Frances Kelsey was dissatisfied with the data submitted by Richardson-Merrell Inc., the American firm that wanted to market the drug. In 1962 thalidomide was banned world-wide.

Dr McBride was awarded a CBE, the Order of Australia and a gold medal from the French Institut de la Vie. He was named Australian Father of the Year in 1972 and was given the Order of Australia in 1977. The money awards provided him with the means of continuing his researches and helped him to set up his Foundation 41 Research Institute in Sydney. Dr McBride became a celebrity and a favourite with the media. He was regularly called on for his comments on medical matters of all kinds. He even helped to advertise American Express Cards.

Full extent of the disaster

The full extent of the disaster did not become clear until the autumn of 1962. It was then admitted by the West German Public Health Ministry that since 1957, when – because of its safety – thalidomide had been approved for over-the-counter sale, it had caused about 10,000 cases of birth malformations in West Germany alone. A great many of these babies had died but about half of them had survived to live with gross deformity and disability. In Britain, there were about 400 surviving malformed children. In Canada, more than 50, and in the USA only a handful. These had resulted from pre-marketing clinical trials. World-wide, there were estimated to be about 10,000 surviving deformed children. The drug had been sold under no fewer than 50 different trade names, many of them mixtures of thalidomide and other drugs – compounds such as Tensival, Valgraine, Valgis, Asmaval, Grippex, Peracon expectorans and Poltgripan. Even after the dangers of thalidomide were known by almost everyone, pregnant women were still taking the drug because they had no idea that it was in the preparation they were using. Everyone knew the name thalidomide, but this did not appear on any of the labels. The adverse publicity – and by now there was plenty of that – more often referred to 'thalidomide' than to any of the many trade names.

The thalidomide tragedy wonderfully concentrated the minds of the pharmaceutical industry and of the various agencies responsible for licensing drugs. Up to this time, few had considered the possible effects of drugs on the early foetus and drugs were not routinely tested for such effects. Now the word 'teratogenicity' (the ability to cause serious developmental errors) was heard everywhere in drug circles. In Britain, the Committee on the Safety of Medicines was set up to monitor and control the production of new drugs. As a result, legislation was introduced to ensure that no new drug could be marketed until independent experts were agreed that it had been adequately tested and was safe. The committee was also concerned to ensure that doctors reported adverse reactions to drugs. The American Food and Drug Administration (FDA) was already performing this function. Where such drug regulatory authorities did not exist, they were now set up all over the world.

Postscript

There is a sad postscript to the thalidomide story. Dr William McBride seemed to be impelled to try to repeat the triumph that had made him world-famous in 1961. Fame can be addictive. Ten years later Dr McBride publicly announced that he had found another drug that could cause birth defects. Apparently, he had discovered an association between the antidepressant drug imipramine, taken by three pregnant women and foetal abnormalities. At once there was a public demand for the banning of the drug. But when Government drug experts interviewed Dr McBride they found that he could provide no evidence of this alleged effect.

In 1980 Dr McBride claimed that he had found yet another drug that produced similar effects on foetuses. The antispasmodic and antihistamine combination drug dicyclomine-doxylamine, marketed by the American company Merrell Dow as Debendox, and used to treat nausea and vomiting in early pregnancy, could, he said, cause deformities in a small percentage of the embryos of women who took it in early pregnancy. Dr McBride appeared as an expert witness in several cases of litigation against Merrell Dow, brought by the parents of congenitally deformed children. Although Merrell Dow denied the charges, the cost of litigation and the bad publicity caused them to withdraw Debendox in 1983.

Dr McBride backed up his opinion about Debendox in a paper he published in the *Australian Journal of Biological Sciences* in 1981. This paper was a study of the drug hyoscine which is chemically related to one of the constituents of Debendox. Two colleagues who had been involved in the research, however, confronted him with the suggestion that he had changed some of the original findings. Various drafts of the manuscript showed progressive changes to the data. His response failed to satisfy them and they resigned from their appointments in his private medical and research foundation. The allegations about Debendox were discredited.

The matter then became public and charges against Dr McBride were laid before a New South Wales medical tribunal. The enquiry took three and a half years and is estimated to have cost £4.5 million. In the course of the enquiry Dr McBride finally admitted that he had published false data. He had done this in the interests of mankind because he was completely convinced that the drug was dangerous. This conviction had allowed him to set aside 'proper scientific principles'. In August 1993, the tribunal reached its conclusion that Dr McBride was guilty of scientific fraud and ordered that he should be struck off the medical register.

This was another thalidomide tragedy. As the tribunal reported, Dr McBride's eminence, good deeds and interest in human welfare, commanded respect and admiration. He was, perhaps, a man by whom the bubble, reputation, was sought just a little too arduously. He had been found guilty of scientific fraud.

Uses of thalidomide

Thalidomide is still a useful drug. It is highly effective in controlling a serious complication of the treatment of leprosy – an unpleasant reaction in which high fever and raised nodules in the skin occur. It is also useful in the treatment of the unpleasant condition of Behçet's syndrome, a persistent disease that causes painful, recurrent ulcers of the mouth and genital area, internal inflammation of the eyes (uveitis), arthritis and blisters, pustules and inflammatory bumps on the skin. Perhaps most important of all, thalidomide seems likely to be effective in preventing a rejection reaction in bone marrow transplantation.

Although it was not until 1961 that the public became generally aware of the question of the proper testing of new drugs, there had, from time to time, been a good deal of professional concern. In the late nineteenth century when chloroform was being increasingly used as a general anaesthetic for surgery, it gradually became clear that this wonderfully pleasant and easy-to-take drug was not as safe as had been thought. After a most promising start, it proved to be so dangerous that between 1879 and 1890 various commissions had to be set up to investigate it.

In 1922 an enquiry was mounted after it was found that many of the patients being treated with the anti-syphilis drug salvarsan were suffering enough liver damage to cause jaundice.

The American Food and Drug Administration was set up after another drug tragedy in 1937. This was the era of the sulpha drugs – the first really effective treatments for internal infections. The then most important member of this drug group, sulphanilamide, was being widely prescribed at this time. The drug itself was reasonably safe although it was known to have some possible side effects on the kidneys and on the blood-forming tissue of the bone marrow. Things really went wrong when a preparation of sulphanilamide was released in the form of a liquid elixir. This drug tasted horrible and it needed a strong-tasting solvent to make it palatable to children. Unfortunately, the solvent chosen for this purpose was the sweet-tasting diethylene glycol. This liquid is very similar to the antifreeze ethylene glycol. It is hardly necessary to say that both of them are highly poisonous.

Sulphanilamide elixir was not tested for safety by its manufacturers. The result was that 107 people died before the medicine was withdrawn. There was, of course, a public outcry, but when the matter was investigated it was found that the firm that produced it had not contravened any law. In 1938 the US Congress passed the Food, Drug and Cosmetic Act and the FDA was born.

Regrettably, until the thalidomide disaster, the idea of testing new drugs for their possible effects on unborn children had, apparently occurred to no one. Some experts have claimed that no one could have foreseen this possibility. This is not quite true. The fact is that prior to the introduction of thalidomide in April 1958, around 400 substances were known to be capable of producing foetal abnormalities in laboratory animals. Certainly, only a few of these substances had ever been used as drugs, but the information did exist.

In sickness, in wealth

The research and testing process for new drugs is highly pressurized, and research scientists are increasingly resorting to fraud. In the past few years a number of now famous cases have come to light.

Dr John Darsee, a research physician who was testing the effects of various heart drugs on dogs with an induced heart condition, and who had already published articles on his work widely, was asked by the head of his department to supply the data on which his latest piece destined for publication was based. This should have consisted of several weeks' monitoring of the dogs' blood flow, heart condition, tissue samples, and so on.

To the amazement of his fellow workers, Darsee promptly dashed back to the laboratory, hooked up a dog to a series of electronic monitors, pumped it full of drugs, and began the experiment he claimed to have been conducting for months. In open view, he began to fabricate the data. As the information on the drug's performance poured out of the machines, Darsee simply re-marked the charts to indicate that this one day's research represented two weeks' work. Darsee had been cheating for the previous seven years, principally in experiments concerning the effectiveness of heart drugs. Darsee's explanation was: 'This was an extremely difficult period for me; I had too much to do, too little time to do it in ... I had put myself on a track that I hoped would allow me to have a wonderful academic job and I knew I had to work very hard for it.'

Rather more notorious is the case of the painted mouse. It is instructive, not only because of the manifest stupidity of the man involved, but of what it implies about the modern research environment.

On 26 March 1974 a flustered young American research scientist, clutching a cage full of mice, found himself alone in an elevator between floors at the prestigious Sloan-Kettering Institute in New York. This research scientist, William Summerlin, was on his way from the laboratory to the director's office to demonstrate the success of his current project.

Summerlin, a highly ambitious young man, had a pressing problem. As the elevator carried him towards the director's office, it propelled his career towards imminent extinction. The problem concerned the mice, which were the wrong colour.

The mice Summerlin was carrying were an integral part of a research programme into the difficulties of human organ transplantation. Without the painstaking medical steps customarily taken to outwit the body's natural immune system, the transplantation of organs from a donor to a recipient would generally be unsuccessful. The only perfect match occurs when the two parties are genetically identical. In the case of animals this requires that they should be from the same inbred strain; in the case of humans, they should be identical twins.

In matching donor organ to recipients, specialists try to obtain the best possible match between what are called HLA or histo-compatibility antigens. These are an individual's cellular signature: they coat each cell of an organism and are genetically determined. The body's immune system recognizes and rejects even minutely foreign HLA, like a banker spotting a fraudulent signature on a cheque. Hence, specialists carefully try to match the signature; but even so, transplants are not universally successful. Any technique or chemical which could make a donor organ acceptable to a recipient, irrespective of the genetic match of the two, could be of enormous commercial value.

One way to do this would be to camouflage the donor organ by weakening or removing some of its HLA; it would then be concealed from the eyes of the body's immune system and could be slipped in without being noticed.

Summerlin had been working on this approach. He had been taking skin grafts from mice, soaking them in various solutions in an attempt to remove some of the identifying HLA, and then grafting the pieces of skin on to other, genetically different mice. He claimed success in transplanting skin from black mice to white mice. If true, this apparently small event was part of a potentially momentous chain of research. Unfortunately, Summerlin had been lying. The skin grafts on the white mice he was carrying were not black.

In the elevator Summerlin did a very strange thing; he took a black felt-tip pen from his pocket, and coloured in the patches of transplanted skin on the white mice. In an instant he had succeeded in producing the vital skin graft that years of research had not yielded.

That afternoon, a laboratory technician discovered that the 'skin grafts' could be washed away with alcohol. It later emerged that claims Summerlin had made for his past work, in which he was said to have successfully transplanted corneas from human cadavers into the eyes of rabbits and adrenal glands from one strain of mice into another, were also fraudulent.

It seems bizarre that a rational, intelligent man could so delude himself as to believe that such fundamental deceit could go undetected indefinitely; or that, in this unlikely event, he would be prepared to live with the potentially serious consequences; what would happen if the research progressed to humans?

In the ensuing public furore of the affair of the painted mouse, it became clear that while Summerlin was principally to blame, he was very much the product of a research environment that required, for prestige and funding from the drug companies, continuous new discoveries.

Summerlin, who had been recently warned by his director that he had failed to produce anything significant of late, had begun to direct his 'research', not towards any scientific end, but towards doing what seemed most expedient – pleasing his employers. His boss was happy to be pleased, and eager to publish the results of experiments before they had been properly verified.

The Opren case

Next to thalidomide, one of the worst single instances of drug-induced death has been the case of Opren. Opren was an arthritis drug aimed at the huge market this chronic illness creates. All anti-inflammatory, non-steroid drugs (like aspirin) are known to cause some side-effects, like internal bleeding. In 1980 Eli Lilley, the producers of Opren, won approval to market the drug in Britain. Their million-pound promotional campaign set out to convince doctors that Opren really was something unique: an arthritis drug which hit at the basis of the disease, stopping the inflammatory process. Furthermore, Opren (the advertisement read) 'had an outstanding gastric tolerance level, in fact the side-effects story [sic] is very impressive indeed, as they are generally mild.'

Opren was only on the US market for a few months, under another name, Oraflex. It was then removed from sale and the company was charged for not alerting the authorities to adverse reactions within the statutory period. Lilley ended up paying $50 million to the US victims of Oraflex/Opren, including one settlement of $6 million to one man whose elderly mother died after taking the drug.

In Britain, the launch of Opren was one of the most successful marketing pushes ever. Within two years, doctors had written nearly a million and a half prescriptions for the drug. But at least seventy, principally elderly, patients died and another estimated 4000 suffered ghastly internal injuries including gastrointestinal bleeding and kidney and liver failure, and sensitivity to light.

Whereas the US financial settlements were at least some retribution and provided a degree of commensurate compensation, Eli Lilley refused to admit liability in Britain. They fought in the courts for five years, and finally the British claimants, some 1300 in number, were driven to settle for a total of £2.75 million, or about £2000 per head, for fear of getting nothing in the end.

Chapter Six

Blunders with the brain

Madmen on show

It is only comparatively recently, it seems, that doctors have felt any real sympathy for mentally disordered people. In the late sixteenth century attitudes to the insane were particularly harsh. This was mainly because of religious dogma that held that such people were inhabited by evil spirits or had decided to accept the blandishments of the Devil. Intolerance to this kind of thing, and hardening attitudes to people who caused trouble, led to the widespread view that the right thing to do with such people was to lock them up and forget about them.

The scenes in psychiatric prisons such as St Mary of Bethlehem (Bedlam) in London were terrible to behold. Official attitudes were explicit. Because the insane were deprived of reason, they were no longer human and should be treated as beasts. They could, of course, be dangerous so were to be closely restrained. Mad people understood physical punishment, however, and could therefore be beaten into submission. They could feel neither heat nor cold and were incapable of feeling shame. Clothes were therefore unnecessary so they were left naked.

It was a popular amusement to visit Bedlam to view the human animals. In the early eighteenth century the authorities made a nice little income from showing off the naked savages. The charge was one penny, and in a single year no fewer than 96,000 spectators attended. £400 a year and practically no overheads. Moreover, this was long-term income. The insane were considered incurable and their incarceration was permanent. Naturally, no one was going to bother to check whether, in fact, any of the inmates actually did recover.

Where it existed, formal medical treatment, even of those not suspected of witchcraft, was not noted for its humanity. In some European centres attempts at treatment, if it can be called that, were made. These were largely at the whim of the doctors. The German psychiatrist Johann Christian Reil (1759–1813), widely regarded as an advanced and humane practitioner, recommended hunger, confinement, flogging with a cowhide, the straitjacket, firing canons and throwing psychiatric patients into cold water in order to bring them to their senses.

Humanitarian advance

In France, however, a notable humanitarian advance was to occur towards the end of the eighteenth century. The French physician Philippe Pinel (1745-1826), in charge of psychiatric patients at the Bicêtre Hospital, at the height of the Reign of Terror, decided that, in some cases, insane behaviour was due to chaining. Pinel, at great risk of dismissal by the authorities for his heretical views, ordered their chains removed. He also allowed certain patients the freedom to move freely around the hospital grounds and to enjoy the fresh air. The experiment was a dramatic success. Many recovered so completely as to be able to be released.

Pinel's successor, Jean-Etiénne Dominique Esquirol (1772-1840) pursued the same policy and was so influential that he was able to have most of the regulations governing the management of the mentally disordered amended. Soon the French ideas spread. Similar reforms were effected in England by members of the distinguished Quaker Tuke family. William Tuke's asylum in Yorkshire became famous for its enlightened treatment of the psychiatrically disordered. In the United States, the Massachusetts schoolteacher, Dorothea Dix was able to achieve similar reforms by bringing the plight of such patients to the notice of the public. Dorothea Dix also campaigned in Europe with considerable success. By the end of the nineteenth century a widespread movement toward more humane treatment of the mentally disordered had been achieved.

Black butterflies

America, 1847: a highly competent and, by all accounts, pleasant manual labourer of Irish extraction named Phineas Gage is involved in rock blasting operations in mountainous terrain. In the course of one sadly uncontrolled explosion, an iron bar is picked up by the force of the blast and driven clean through the front part of his head. Phineas is sent flying, but to everybody's surprise he is not dead, and survives the removal of the protruding bar. As he recovers, however, it is observed that his personality has dramatically changed, though his memory and intelligence remain apparently unaffected. In 1868, a physician named Harlow from Boston writes about him: 'His equilibrium, or balance, so to speak, between his intellectual faculties and animal propensities seems to have been destroyed. He is fitful, irreverent, indulging in the grossest profanity (which was not previously his custom), manifesting but little deference for his fellows, impatient of restraint or advice when it conflicts with his desires.' The now extremely rude Phineas Gage is an object of immense medical interest, for it seems clear, from his somewhat crude experience of psychosurgery, that one can alter the social behaviour of the human animal by physically interfering with the frontal lobes of the brain.

Dr Gottlieb Burckhardt

In 1890, Dr Gottlieb Burckhardt, the superintendent of a psychiatric hospital in Switzerland, drills holes in the heads of six severely agitated patients and extracts sections of the frontal lobes, altering their behaviour with varying degrees of success. Two of the patients die. His surgery is considered morally reprehensible at the time, but his work is not forgotten.

Phineas and his iron bar have started a train of thought that will come to a strange and tragic fruition in the next century.

In the aftermath of the First World War, America was suffering from a huge increase in psychiatric disorders. An influx of shell-shocked soldiers and bereaved, disturbed relatives was swelling the asylum population. In addition, there was still no cure for tertiary syphilis, which had been discovered to cause up to half the known cases of dementia praecox, or schizophrenia. People were still poisoning syphilis-sufferers with a mixture of mercury, bismuth, iodides, and arsenic compounds.

Dr William White and Dr Walter Freeman

At George Washington University the Professor of Psychiatry, Dr William White, a man with a firm belief in the need for strong, therapeutic intervention in this psychiatric crisis, met a young and popular neurologist named Walter Freeman, whose theatrically compelling lectures at the university were so engrossing that students would bring their girlfriends along in preference to going to the cinema. Born in Philadelphia in 1895, the son of a doctor with strong Calvinist beliefs, Freeman had a ferocious work ethic.

Freeman was soon appointed Professor of Neurology. Inspired by the example of his grandfather, an adventurous and successful surgeon who pioneered the use of brain surgery to remove tumours, Freeman specialized in the relatively young study of nervous diseases. But his early experiences of American psychiatric hospitals, with their slouching figures, vacantly staring, or gibbering inmates, and general shabbiness filled him, by his own confession, with a mixture of fear, disgust and shame. He felt inadequate and helpless. He could not empathize with the inmates; he was repelled by them. In the absence of any clear, simple medical way to treat patients, he retreated to his first loves, the laboratory, and the lecture room.

White and Freeman got on well, which is not that usual among psychiatrists and neurologists. They talked about the need for practical measures to counter at least syphilis-induced madness. Freeman was impressed by White's belief in physical intervention in mental disorder. Most psychiatrists didn't hold with that. White heard about the work of Julius Wagner-Jauregg in Vienna, who had been using infected blood derived from a malaria-crazed soldier to perform shock therapy on syphilis sufferers. The malaria raised the body temperature so high that the syphilis microbes were (in theory) destroyed.

White had a dozen malaria-carrying mosquitoes shipped to America in a tiny cage. Unfortunately, eleven died in transit, having become stuck to an exposed strip of sticky tape. The precious surviving mosquito was placed in a tiny meshed cage and strapped to the wrist of a man suffering from dementia praecox induced by tertiary syphilis. The man had been insane for years, and had in the course of speculative treatments inhaled so much mercury that his innards had rotted and he was near death anyway. After infection with malaria, his temperature soared as the fever ravaged and crippled his body, pushing him to the uttermost limits of life. But the fever finally subsided, and although the results were obscure as the man remained delirious, it could be supposed that this dramatic, and painful strike at the roots of mental illness had achieved some good.

The man died a few days later of a number of complications. But Freeman found the experience highly impressive. For him, it intimated that one was not helpless in the face of acute psychiatric disorder; one was not simply stuck with abstract cures like psychoanalysis, or endless warm baths, which he thought futile. There must be a means, no matter how drastic, of tackling madness physically.

Freeman meets Pavlov and Egas Moniz

In July 1935 Walter Freeman, now forty years old, and slowly recovering from the nervous breakdown recently precipitated by overwork, was in London, where he had gone to attend a neurological conference. It was quite a gathering. Also in attendance was the celebrated Russian Ivan Pavlov, whose trained, salivating dogs (which he did not bring with him) were to make him legendary. In addition, Freeman discovered that he had set up his stall just down the hallway from Egas Moniz, a Portuguese aristocrat, former ambassador to Spain, and

Portugal's signatory to the Versailles Treaty. Moniz was also a celebrated neurosurgeon, having pioneered cerebral angiography, the process of mapping the parts of the brain by injecting 'contrast' solutions which can be seen by X-rays. Freeman could not help being a little jealous of the kindly old gentleman, then sixty-one years old. He, Freeman sighed, had made his great discovery and could now rest on his laurels. Great discoveries were important to Freeman.

Pavlov might not have brought his dogs to the conference, but John Fulton from Yale University had brought two chimpanzees. These were the subject of a day-long symposium which both Freeman and Moniz attended. Fulton had completely removed the entire frontal lobes from these two animals – a lobectomy – which had radically altered their behaviour. He could no longer generate experimental forms of neurosis in the animals. They were placid, indeed, seemingly unperturbable. The symposium was fascinated, and the discussion about the significance of the frontal lobes went on and on, as the assembled company hedged gently around the delicate issue that Fulton's chimpanzees raised. Eventually, to much surprise, it was Egas Moniz who stood up, and asked the question that Freeman, for one, had been desperate to put.

'If the frontal lobe removal prevents the development of experimental neurosis in animals and eliminates frustrational behaviour,' he asked, 'why would it not be possible to relieve anxiety states in man by surgical means?'

Many attending were shocked to hear it put so frankly; they believed that Moniz was talking about performing the full lobectomy on humans. Two months after the London conference, in the autumn of 1935, Moniz was back in Portugal, about to participate in an event which would have a profound effect on the lives of hundreds of thousands throughout the world.

Operating on the brain

In a Lisbon surgery, a patient from a local asylum, the Manicomio Bombarda, a woman with a history of anxiety, melancholy and hypochondria, was lying, heavily anaesthetized and with her head shaved, on a table. She was strapped to it but, curiously, she was not flat; her torso propped up at a 45-degree angle by the special contours of the table, and there was a sandbag behind her neck which pushed her head upright. This posture was accentuated by canvas tethers, which pulled the naked skull forwards. Her gown was very securely fastened; everything that might move was restrained, as if the operation were known to be one of such finesse, such delicacy, that the slightest twitch or reaction would jeopardize it.

On the small stand next to the operating table were three curious objects: a syringe with a long needle; a bottle of alcohol; and an instrument with a short shaft, at one end of which was a small circle of sharp metal teeth and at the other a spike-like handle.

There were two surgeons present. One was Egas Moniz. Despite his skill and experience, Moniz did not trust his hands not to shake with age, and the gout from which he suffered, and had employed the services of a much younger man to assist him. This was Almeida Lima, a brilliant neurosurgeon, and a man who, like Moniz, was fascinated by the thought processes that define the human.

Together, the surgeons scrubbed the cranium of the drugged and restrained woman with a caustic, antiseptic cocktail of soap, water, iodine, ether, and alcohol. Then, using gentian violet, a colouring derived from crystal and methyl violet, they drew on the pale skin of the patient's head. Under instruction from Moniz, the young Lima sketched two lines, one extending across the top of the head, from ear to ear, and one dividing the head down the middle. They had visually quartered the brain underneath the bone of the skull, and these lines provided a crude map for what was to follow. The two surgeons were attempting to perform the first leucotomy. They did not want to destroy the actual frontal lobes, but rather to destroy the fibres, the white matter or leukos, which connect the frontal lobes, those areas they believed to be most immediately concerned with social behaviour, to the main body of the human brain. They were going to try to cure madness by disconnecting the frontal lobes from the parts of the brain that they thought might be exerting a disturbing influence on them. They were pulling the plug on the patient's emotions.

Lima made incisions in the skin, on both sides of the head, at points about an inch and a half either side of the purple central dividing line and, viewed from above, an inch and a half in front of the ears. He pulled back the skin. Moniz whispered to Lima that the incisions looked like a strange pair of slanted eyes; indeed, they seemed to stare accusingly at the young neurosurgeon.

Lima took the peculiar instrument with the sharp teeth and used it to cut into the bone of the skull that his incisions had exposed. Within minutes, two little rondels of bone were extracted from the head and placed in a tray. The two men, though very tense, were increasingly excited, and gave each other reassuring smiles; have courage, said Moniz, and all will be well.

The two holes in the skull revealed the pulsating, delicate

grey of the brain, supported and shielded by muscular, complex sheathing, floating miraculously on a bed of shining cerebrospinal fluid. Millions of glittering, microscopic neural pathways snaked out from the top of the spinal cord, looking like the roots of a tree, and entwined themselves in the higher regions of the brain, merging into a soft, gelatinous, confused, and utterly mysterious mass, among which are entrapped and dispersed the very secrets of who we are.

Lima gently swabbed the visible areas with an antiseptic saline solution; anything stronger would damage the brain, perhaps even destroying some of the tissue. The words of Moniz flickered through Lima's mind. 'To cure these patients we must destroy,' Moniz had said; but he wanted to destroy selectively, to explore the possibility of excising the fugitive, elusive afflictions of the mind. If mental sickness, so disparate, so frustrating to the rational being, could be found to be localized in a region of the mind in the same way as physical illnesses have their seats in other organs – the heart, the stomach, the pancreas, and the liver – then perhaps it might be possible to chop it out, and toss it away, like a tumour.

Moniz handed Lima the long-needled syringe. It contained two cubic centimetres of alcohol, which would be injected to destroy brain matter.

Lima pushed the needle of the syringe through one of the exploratory apertures, down through the protective sheathing, down into the brain, and then sharply shoved it forward two inches into the frontal cortex, and through, penetrating the network of neural fibres, that junction box of white matter, behind the forehead. He injected the alcohol which began immediately to disperse throughout the tissue, to dissolve and irreparably destroy the fibres. Some indefinable element of the personality quietly died, the spidery, infinitesimally delicate wires of the neural connections reduced to a grey fluid. Lima pulled the needle out. As he did so, the needle inevitably sucked alcohol up with it, back into the actual frontal-lobe cortex, killing millions of cells; it was a problem they had anticipated, but things would be easier when the special knife arrived. Lima repeated the process on the other side of the head. Then it was all over – for this patient, anyway: Lima and Moniz had another three waiting to experiment on.

Results

After surgery, the woman was certainly less agitated, overtly paranoid and disturbed than she had been before; but she and the other three patients from the asylum who underwent the same procedure were also, Moniz admitted, somewhat more apathetic and frankly dull than he had hoped, and suffered from nausea, sphincter disorders, sheer sluggishness and disorientation. Still, the results were spectacular enough for Moniz to be enormously encouraged. Unfortunately, he also found that the director of the asylum, seeing that the immediate results Moniz was obtaining with his experimental surgery made his years of fruitless treatment seem rather redundant, was suffering twinges of professional jealousy and was unwilling to supply any more surgical subjects. Quite apart from this, he was, as Lima put it, experiencing 'doctrinal and ethical' doubts about the nature of the operation. In order to maintain his flow of patients, therefore, Moniz not only had to exercise his considerable powers of charm, but began to withhold the results of his work that suggested it was less than perfect, so that it appeared that the operation was already a success, and one so simple that it could be quickly applied on a wide, public basis.

From its beginning, psychosurgery was synonymous with deception.

The knife was a success. Moniz kept his work secret, to avoid the widespread pirating of his technique. When he did publish his results, it was in six countries simultaneously. Hence, as one contemporary said of this extraordinary phenomenon, 'Seldom in the history of medicine has an experimental procedure been so promptly adapted to the treatment of sick patients everywhere.'

World-wide acceptance of lobotomy

It did take a few years, and the work of a faithful band of pioneers, to establish the various forms of lobotomy as everyday treatment for psychiatric patients, but by 1955 over 40,000 men, women and children in the United States alone had undergone psychosurgery which left large parts of their brains irreparably vandalized by doctors who didn't even need a formal qualification to practice the operation.

The greatest advocate of psychosurgery was Walter Freeman. In June 1936 he came across Moniz's first, brief article on the leucotomy in a French medical periodical, and immediately requested a copy of Moniz's full monograph on the process from its Paris publisher. Although he was a neurologist, Freeman had no qualifications as a surgeon. He needed a neurosurgeon as a collaborator. He showed the book to his neurosurgeon colleague, James Watts. They ordered two of Moniz's leucotomes from France, and then went on a holiday.

On their return to their Washington base, the knives had arrived; and, moreover, a mere year after that London conference, Freeman received from Moniz an autographed copy of his work. It was an inspiration. After a week of practicing on brains from the morgue, Freeman and Watts operated on their first living patient. Watts did the cutting; Freeman navigated.

More 'progress'

She was a sixty-three-year-old woman from Kansas, the type of agitated, depressed and fearful personality that Moniz had experimented on. Faced with a choice of a mental institution or surgery, she and her husband opted for the knife. On the operating table, she had second thoughts when she realized that her head was about to be shaved, and she would lose the curls that she was proud of. Freeman assured her that her curls would be saved; this was not the case, but after the operation, as Freeman himself noted, 'She no longer cared'.

The operation was carried out on 14 September 1936. Moniz had altered his prescribed technique since the first leucotomy, and six holes were now cut in the patient's head. When she had been stitched together and had awoken from the anaesthetic, the sense of calm she exuded in contrast with her former terror was striking, even weird. When asked by Freeman if she could remember why she had previously been so upset, she could only say: 'I don't know. I seem to have forgotten. It doesn't seem important now.' She smiled beatifically at her husband, and rose to meet him as he entered the surgery.

Freeman and Watts were thrilled by the results.

A week after surgery, the woman began to behave strangely. She talked incoherently, becoming stuck on certain syllables, repeating them endlessly and hopelessly jumbling up her sentences. She could no longer recite the days of the week, and when she was asked to write, the same repetitions, and sad, nonsensical constructions occurred on paper. A few days later, her speech had principally returned and she went placidly home, showing neither eagerness nor apprehension.

The two surgeons proceeded to operate on another five patients over the next six weeks, and in November 1936 published a report in which they wrote: 'In all our patients there was a ... common denominator of worry, apprehension, anxiety, insomnia and nervous tension, and in all of them these particular symptoms have been relieved to a greater or lesser extent.' They further said that in some patients disorientation, confusion, phobias, hallucinations, and delusions had been relieved or had altogether disappeared. They concluded by stating the grounds on which they had undertaken the operations – to relieve symptoms that were causing 'great distress to the patients and to their families '– and added: 'We wish to emphasize that indiscriminate use of the procedure could result in vast harm. Prefrontal [targeted at the parts of the brain behind the frontal lobes] leucotomy should at present be reserved for a small group of specially selected cases ... every patient probably loses something by this operation, some spontaneity, some sparkle, some flavour of the personality, if it may be so described.'

They were publicly more cautious than Moniz, dismissing thoughts of instant cures. Privately, however, Freeman was triumphant. Talking about their first patient, he said: 'This woman went back home in ten days, and she is cured.' The 'indiscriminate use' he and Watts counselled against would come, irrespective of their warnings; Freeman himself would provide the means, and the motivation for it.

Freeman and Watts considered that leucotomy was an incorrect name for the procedure. It suggested that it was only the white matter, the leukos, that was affected. They saw that they also destroyed actual nerve cells. Hence, they renamed it the lobotomy. This also helped to establish their version of the operation as distinct from that performed by Moniz. They were now the pioneers.

Changes of strategy

They began to perceive the limitations of the current mode of operation: eight of their initial twenty patients had two operations, and two of these had a third; there were two fatalities. Soon they were trying variations on the theme. They tried it with more holes in the top of the head, and penetrated deeper. They substituted for the cutting wire of the leucotome a more rigid blade, but found that the blade frequently broke off in the patient's brain, and when it could eventually be dragged out, bits of blood vessel and brain tissue came with it.

By 1938, Freeman decided to change the strategy for attacking the brain. He opted to make the holes in the side of the head, to allow a more direct assault on the white matter. He also changed the instrument to a narrow steel blade, blunt and flat like a butter knife, called a Killian periosteal elevator. In principle, the blunt, thin end of this could be gently pushed through the intervening brain tissue with less risk of tearing the blood vessels.

From this development emerged the 'Freeman-Watts standard lobotomy' – or, as they called it, the 'precision method'. After hand-drilling holes on either side of the head which were widened by manually breaking away further bits of the skull, the way would be paved for the knife by the preliminary insertion of a six-inch cannula, the tubing from a heavy-gauge hypodermic needle. Put in one hole, this would be aimed at the other on the opposite side of the head. Then the blunt knife was inserted in the path initially carved by the cannula. Once inside the brain, the blade was swung in two cutting arcs, destroying the targeted nerve matter. 'It goes through just like soft butter,' said Watts. The operation was repeated on the other side.

Blind operations

Because the technique was 'blind' – they could not see what they were doing – it required both men. Watts manipulated the cannula and blade while Freeman, who habitually chewed spruce gum throughout operations, crouched in front of the patient, like a baseball catcher, using his knowledge of the internal map of the brain to give Watts instructions such as 'up a bit', 'down a fraction', or 'straight ahead'. Watts enjoyed 'flying on instruments only', as he put it, and became so expert that as a special trick, he could insert a cannula through a two-millimetre hole in one side of a patient's head and thread it through the brain, and out of the opposing minute hole like a shoelace. 'That's pretty damn dramatic, you know,' he once said. 'And of course it always impressed spectators.' Viewers were stunned by the sight of a man with a tube apparently passing straight through his brain.

The best was yet to come. Having observed that the optimum results were achieved when the lobotomy induced drowsiness and disorientation, Freeman and Watts decided to see if they could use this information to judge how an operation was proceeding; they began to perform lobotomies under local anaesthetic. Now they could speak to the patient while cutting the lobe connections and gauge whether they were being successful. They asked patients to sing a song, or to perform arithmetic, and if they could see no signs of disorientation, they chopped away some more until they could.

Initial professional reaction to the 1936 operations was not promising. Although, privately, the technique aroused great interest, it drew outraged responses from psychoanalysts and many psychiatrists, though in keeping with the medical tradition of discretion, these reservations were not voiced to the public at the time. Ten years later, everybody would declare that they had always opposed the lobotomy.

Professional reactions

Freeman's presentations to the profession were sourly received. Critics referred to the 'offhand manner' in which the operation was described. Dr Lewis Polack, angered by Freeman's manipulation of public opinion via the press, said to his face that it was 'immoral to offer to the public any sort of a procedure which would awaken expectation and hope without possible fulfilment ... it is not an operation, but a mutilation ... there are different sizes of skulls and brains and there is no way of knowing what may be removed.' Freeman, buoyed up by the enthusiasm he had aroused in the popular press, was by his own admission 'dogmatic and provocative'.

For the time being, he and Watts could not obtain the access they coveted to the many thousands of inmates of asylums. 'It'll be a hell of a long time before you operate on any of my patients,' said one asylum director to Freeman. They remained in Washington, doing what work they could.

Once the initial revulsion had been expressed, more measured noises were made. An influential psychiatrist, Adolf Meyer, gave a cautious welcome to the lobotomy, and a respected medical journal concluded that 'the operation is based ... on sound physiological observations and is a much more rational procedure than many that have been suggested in the past for the surgical relief of mental disease.' One of this journal's editorial board was none other than John Fulton, the man whose chimpanzees had aroused Moniz's interest; he may even have written the article himself.

The introduction and wide acceptance around this time of other shock therapies such as metrazol (the fear drug), sodium amytal (the truth drug) and insulin-coma shock therapy began to create a climate in which the lobotomy might seem more acceptable. Freeman was a neurologist, a specialist in the study of nervous diseases, and neurologists had traditionally taken the view that there were physical (organic) causes for mental illness, and that it required physical (organic or somatic) treatment. Psychiatrists, on the other hand, had argued that mental disorder was a problem of the mind exclusively. The two groups had bickered over whose property madness was, and the psychiatrists were initially Freeman's greatest opponents. But in the face of soaring mental hospital populations and the lack of rapid cures, both sides in this bizarre dispute began to adopt increasingly extreme therapies. Overcrowding and limited mental health budgets would finally persuade the superintendents of mental institutions to adopt lobotomy. The economic arguments would be very strong: a lobotomy could be performed for $250, while it could cost $35,000 or more a year to maintain a patient in hospital.

Ironically, all the objections to the lobotomy's acceptance – its drastic nature, the fact that no one understood what it was really doing, its speed as an operation, and the fact that it changed patients (indeed, it recreated them anew in some way) – were turned upside down and inside out and became the reasons for its wide adoption. The psychiatrists could argue that brain surgery did not show that mental disorder had its roots in a disease; and the neurologists could argue that the operation showed that physical intervention, not words, brought about the cure. The lobotomy was a convenient means of settling a number of conflicts.

Popular reaction to lobotomy

Freeman, as noted earlier, was a great lecturer, and to overcome the initial professional prejudice against the operation, he travelled tirelessly and gave presentations across the nation. He was also a skilful manipulator of the media; his ability to go over the heads of his medical colleagues, and communicate directly with the public was a crucial asset. His work made excellent copy. In 1936, before Freeman had even disclosed details of his first operations to his professional colleagues, he had lunch with a reporter from the Washington *Evening Star*, whom he had asked if he 'wanted to see some history made. We've done a few brain operations on crazy people with interesting results.' The reporter was also given a chance to see the two men in action, and within a few days Freeman and Watts were on the front page of the *New York Times*, their technique – barely tried, unproven, and already with some dubious results – was hailed as a 'shining example of therapeutic courage.'

Thereafter, Freeman cultivated particular relationships with popular journalists, and fed them tasty copy, eschewing the customary routes of the medical press to publicize his work. He featured on the front page of the *New York Times* and other national dailies and periodicals regularly over the following years, undoubtedly persuading many surgeons to adopt the technique, and many thousands of patients and relatives of patients to opt for it.

The popular coverage was universally optimistic, with headlines such as, 'Surgery Used On The Soul-Sick; Relief Of

Obsessions Is Reported', 'Psychosurgery Cured Me', 'Surgeon's Knife Restores Sanity To Nerve Victims', 'Wizardry Of Surgery Restores Sanity To Fifty Raving Maniacs', 'Forgetting Operation Bleaches Brain', and, memorably, and tragically incorrectly, 'No Worse Than Removing Tooth'.

A sanitized version of the operation, and its consequences was invariably given, never more so than in an influential article entitled, 'Turning The Mind Inside Out', published in the *Saturday Evening Post* in 1941, and considered by Freeman to be a 'brilliant exposition of a very difficult subject.' The writer, the science editor of the *New York Times*, began in dramatic fashion by stating that there must be at least two hundred men and women in the United States who have had worries, persecution complexes, suicidal intentions, obsessions, indecisiveness, nervous tensions literally cut out of their minds with a knife. Freeman had explained the operation to the writer, Waldemar Kaempffert, as one which separated the pre-frontal lobes, 'the rational brain', from the thalamic brain, 'the emotional brain', and the writer warmed to his theme, saying: 'Man must balance emotion and reason. According to the Freeman-Watts theory, the preservation of that balance is a matter of nicely adjusting the "thalamic" feeling with prefrontal logic.' It made it sound disarmingly simple, the brain no more complex than the innards of a watch or a radio with bad reception which could be adjusted by selective use of a screwdriver. The word 'irreversible' was avoided.

Taking Freeman on oath, Kaempffert wrote that the decision to perform the operation was not made lightly, but only after 'careful psychological tests, heart to heart talks with wives, husbands, business associates, and close relatives.' There were in fact no useful psychological tests, and background research on the patients was restricted to a glance at any available medical records and a brief, explanatory chat with whoever had accompanied the patient to the surgery. The article said that Freeman declined to operate on the criminally insane, and believed that a modicum of anxiety was not only normal but desirable. Community life would be impossible if we were not afraid of the police, afraid of upbraidings from our wives and husbands,' said Freeman. It concluded with a vision of spiritual release and earthly contentment: 'We want a little indifference, a little laziness, a little joy of living that patients have sought in vain for so long," says Doctor Freeman. Though the operation may occasionally transform a morbidly anxious man into a happy drone, Doctor Freeman thinks it is better to do so than go through life in an agony of hate and fear of persecution.'

A 'happy drone' indeed.

'Black butterflies' – Freeman's own mental state
In 1941, and laid up in bed with a heavy dose of what he terms influenza, Freeman was still working, correcting the galley proofs of the book that he and Watts had spent the last year putting together. It was called *Psychosurgery: Intelligence, Emotion, and Social Behaviour.* Freeman had done the majority of work for the book, and as ever had ploughed himself into the ground, running a punishing schedule in which he had for months been rising at four in the morning to write for three hours before conducting a full day of clinical work, and teaching at George Washington University. The others involved in the book were quite glad to see him out of the way for a few days, because he had harried them remorselessly to get the project finished and published.

The last time he ran a comparable schedule it precipitated a nervous breakdown, six years beforehand. He was very scared by his own lurch into black depression, and ever since then had taken at least three capsules of Nembutal every night to guarantee sleep. Nembutal also gave him a dreamless sleep. Freeman did not like his dreams.

His depression had deepened his prejudice against personal introspection; he believed that there was nothing to be gained from self-examination except pessimism. He himself was a great believer in activity and exercise. He went off vigorously walking whenever possible, and often prescribed the same remedy for depressed patients. Trying to talk to them was nonsense. Something that had always been a perverse source of amusement to him was the number of psychoanalysts who committed suicide. He could not help pointing out with a certain amount of glee that no fewer than eight of Freud's associates killed themselves. While sitting in bed, looking at the proofs of his new book, an idea for another came into his head: one day he would write a book about these masters of introspection, whose tortured self-concern led only to self-destruction.

He wasn't a great one for personal talk. Although he was a fine communicator, a humorous and often generous man, he seemed to brush personal problems aside. He was afraid of the pauses in conversation, the uncomfortable gaps, the frightening ambiguities of people. He'd never been very comfortable with emotional matters. His mother once called him 'the cat who walks by himself': then a child slightly removed, aloof; now a man in a hurry, evading something inside himself.

Freeman doodled in the corner of the proofs. He drew a skull. He put a crack in it. He remembered his own depression, and felt a spasm of fear, which he clouted to one side, brusquely. He refused to consider that he might be feeling a little off colour. But the sensation of helplessness in the presence of a dark-winged cloud persisted. From the days when he once studied in Paris, a phrase was cast up by his memory.

'J'ai des papillons noirs.'

I have black butterflies. That was how they described depression.

Over the crack in the skull he had drawn, Freeman sketched the dark wings of a storm cloud of black butterflies which, released from the skull, were spiralling upwards, returning to the realm of the spirits. He enlarged the crack into a hole, a drilled hole, like the ones the ancient Inca doctors used to make in the head to allow the evil of madness to escape.

The black butterflies with their huge haunting wings and the skull appeared on the cover of *Psychosurgery*. They provided a dramatic, magical, and fearful image which added a layer of strange superstition to the subject. In addition, Freeman wrote some very snappy and upbeat copy for the covers. 'Read the last chapter to find out how those treasured frontal lobes, supposed to be man's most precious possession, can bring him to suicide and psychosis,' exhorted the dustjacket. It claimed that the volume 'inaugurates a new era in the treatment of mental disorders, a surgical era ... this work reveals how personality can be cut to measure, sounding a note of hope for those who are afflicted with insanity.'

'Cut to measure': Freeman already saw wider applications than those he first cautiously espoused.

Psychosurgery was a considerable success. Lobotomy began to gain in popularity in the United States, though in Europe its acceptance was more limited. Basing their work on the

Freeman-Watts system, American neurosurgeons rapidly developed a myriad of variations. It was five years since Moniz's first operation, and there had still been no long-term study of those who had undergone surgery.

Up until 1945, Freeman had never actually performed a lobotomy himself. He had always worked in tandem with Watts, and his surgical experience was limited to performing 'spinal taps'.

What was still lacking, for Freeman, was a version of the operation that could be performed not just by neurosurgeons, but by anyone, anywhere, in a few minutes: an off-the-peg, rapid technique, so that one could pop down to the local psychiatrist, and get lobotomized in the lunch-break.

Amarro Fiamberti and trans-orbital lobotomy

He had heard of the work of an Italian called Amarro Fiamberti, who had developed a trans-orbital attack on the frontal lobes; one that went in through the front of the skull, directly over the eyeball. He had perforated the orbital plate of the skull behind the eyes, and injected caustic solutions to destroy the brain tissue, but these had sunk down and caused rather severe damage elsewhere. Fiamberti had also punctured the orbital plate directly through the eye sockets and tried to use the original leucotome in this method with few good results, and a lot of mess.

The potential advantage of such an approach was that it did not require holes to be made in the skull; everything could, in theory, be performed by one individual administering a simple stab through the back of each eye socket into the white matter of the brain. There would be nothing to set up. The patient would be left with nothing worse than black eyes and a splitting headache. Plus the usual effects. It would be very easy, very fast, and very cheap.

During the winter of 1945, Freeman tried to develop a trans-orbital approach to lobotomy, practicing on corpses. Watts co-operated, believing that ultimately he would do the surgery, and Freeman would, as usual, navigate.

The two men came up against a familiar problem; the instruments they were using were not strong enough to penetrate the orbital bone, and kept breaking off inside the head of their experimental corpses. They needed an implement that was slender, sharp, and strong.

One day, while mulling over the problem at home, Freeman remembered that the apple-corer had been a source of inspiration for Moniz, and began to rummage through the contents of his kitchen drawers. Soon he found precisely what he was looking for: a cheap, mass-produced ice pick for stabbing pieces of ice off large commercial blocks. Normally essential for making cold drinks on long, hot summer days, it now made its debut as an instrument for brain-surgery. Thank heavens the Kenwood Chef and Magimix had not yet been invented.

Freeman put a special hammer-shaped head on the ice pick, which allowed it to be pushed and pulled more easily. It was used in the first trans-orbital lobotomies in America. The trans-orbital also became known as the 'ice-pick' lobotomy. Curiously, one of Freeman's most vivid childhood memories was a moment when, lying in bed, he saw the head of a pick-axe driven accidentally, but with tremendous force, through the wall of his bedroom.

Armed with his new weapon, Freeman was convinced that a trans-orbital would be a simple piece of surgery which would not require a neurosurgeon. He decided that he would operate on the first living patient without telling Watts, whom he hoped would be enough impressed to offer his encouragement there-after. Secretly, he tried his hand on a series of patients, to whom he explained that the technique had been used success-fully in Italy for a number of years, which was being economi-cal with the truth. He did not dwell on his own lack of surgical experience. He anaesthetized them with three rapid bursts of electric shock. He then drew the upper eyelid away from the eyeball, exposing the tear duct. The sharp point of the ice pick was placed in this, and then, as Freeman put it, 'a light tap with a hammer is usually all that is needed to drive the point through the orbital plate.' The ice pick was plunged into the brain. When it was about two inches inside, Freeman would pull the ice pick about thirty degrees backward, as far as he could without cracking the skull, and then move it up and down in another twenty degree arc, in order to cut the nerves at the base of the frontal lobes. The procedure took only a few minutes. Freeman's post-operative advice to relatives was restricted to the order: 'buy them some sunglasses'.

Freeman and Watts part company

By patient number ten, he felt confident enough to invite Watts along. Watts was not happy to find out what Freeman had been doing, and was deeply distressed to see the perfunctory, brutal nature of the operation. He angrily threatened to break with Freeman if he continued. It was the beginning of the end of their relationship, and within months Watts had left the joint practice they ran. Freeman, now with an incessant itch for surgery, started to sneak off out of Washington, to mental hospitals in other states where he could practice his technique. But he was continually angered by finding himself given the most deteriorated patients to operate on. He wanted trans-orbital lobotomy to be performed on people just developing signs of mental disorder.

The year 1947 brought personal tragedy for Freeman. While walking in Yosemite National Park with his five sons, he saw one of them, the eleven-year-old, Keen, go to the edge of the Vernal Falls on the Merced River to fill a canteen. He fell in, and both he, and the young sailor who tried to save him were swept away by the swollen river and drowned before Freeman's eyes. The bodies were found several days later. Coping with the death was especially difficult for Freeman, who found it impossible to talk about such emotive matters. In his inability to address these he was, though he would have resented the assertion, following a family trait. He had never been communicative with his mother, and when, as a child, he had been caught playing truant, and dragged before his father, instead of receiving the punishment he expected, Freeman had been horrified to see his father take a small cat-o'-nine-tails from his desk, and beat himself on the back until he bled. All emotion, all anger, and the blind, black rage that many suspected was within Freeman were turned inwards, and when they emerged, it was in strange and grotesque fashion. Once he advised a frail woman who consulted him with terrible psychosomatic pains to adopt a heavy routine of exercise and weightlifting. Her original persona was not restored, but utterly changed, destroyed even. She became something new, and something that she was naturally not: a muscle-bound freak. Freeman was proud of the shocking change he had induced and exhibited her photograph.

The following year, 1948, was a much better one for Freeman. He was elected president of the American Board of Psychiatry and Neurology; he drove an expensive Lincoln convertible. Royalties and fees from the operation were making him wealthy. The Freeman-Watts standard lobotomy had been performed on as many as 20,000 disturbed, and not quite so disturbed, individuals worldwide. The end of the Second World War had brought thousands of traumatized veterans back to join those still suffering from the effects of the First World War. In gratitude for their services, they were given shock treatment and psychosurgery.

Freeman was a celebrity whose work was rarely out of the papers. He took advantage of his status to push his trans-orbital technique into the public eye, so to speak, even exhibit-ing it on television to general amazement. The ice pick lobotomy grew in popularity, particularly among psychiatrists without any previous experience of surgery.

In 1948, Walter Freeman performed his most famous trans-orbital lobotomy when he hammered his ice pick into the head of the movie star and radical political activist Frances Farmer. She had rebelled all her life against every form of authority, and despite her success in Hollywood, and on Broadway, found herself incarcerated in the Western State Hospital in Fort Stellacoombe, Washington, aged only thirty-four. The hospital, notorious for its dreadful conditions, institutional violence, rape, and the regular punishment of uncooperative patients with vast doses of electro-shock therapy, had in desperation performed an increasing number of lobotomies on its inmates. Frances Farmer was a particularly sore point, because no treat-ment yet devised seemed to work on her; she would not be tamed. But her openly communist sympathies, and aggression towards officialdom had offended too many people for them to give up without 'curing' her.

Hither rode Walter Freeman, knight to the rescue, ice pick in one hand, hammer in the other. On an October morning, in front of an eager audience of staff, curious visiting psychiatrists, and photographers, female patients in wheelchairs were ranged before the great showman of psychosurgery. After giving a brief lecture to the assembled crowd on the wonders of the ice pick lobotomy – no more complex than a shot of penicillin, no scar, amazing potential for controlling society's misfits, viz, schizophrenics, homosexuals, communists, etc. (Freeman was always quick to seize on new selling points for his art) – he went to work.

Patient number one was wheeled before him. He put the electrodes on her temples and shocked her into a faint, lifted her left eyelid, and plunged the ice pick into her head. He pulled it out. Another women was brought before him. Again he shocked, and stabbed. And another, and then again another, and so on, and on, remorselessly, in a production line of controlled, casual violence until even the director of the hospital, near to passing out with nausea, left the room.

Afterwards, in a dark and silent ward, the patients lay supine on beds, or cried quietly; their faces were disfigured with a questioning blankness. The personality that was Frances Farmer had been effectively terminated earlier in the day, in a remote room to avoid publicity. She was reduced to a state of turgid, generalized mediocrity by the surgery. Society had won its battle with her; she would never again be a threat. An embarrassment, she was released, and, grown fat, and slow, she drifted off into oblivion, and ended her life as a clerk in a hotel, dying of cancer in 1970. Freeman had a photograph of himself performing the lobotomy on her, and, before lobotomy fell into disgrace, he used to show it proudly to friends. In the end, he didn't mention the operation in his memoirs.

People often fainted when watching Walter Freeman at his peak in the late 1940s and early 1950s. Even the eminent Dr Edwin Zabriskie, a seventy-four-year-old who had been involved in bitter hand-to-hand fighting in the First World War, and was a clinical professor of neurology, was seen to crumple on to the carpet at the sight of Freeman, and his trusty ice pick in action.

Though he toured widely throughout America in 1949, Freeman not only taught through live demonstrations, but also made several films, which helped swell the number of operations performed, particularly in the overcrowded hospitals in poorer areas of the country. Within eight months in 1949, 515 trans-orbital lobotomies were performed in Texas alone. At Rusk State Hospital in Texas, where Freeman had made an inspiring personal appearance early in Spring, they were already planning another 450 ice pick lobotomies before the year was out, even though the staff featured no surgeon of any description, only three psychologists and a couple of doctors.

In addition to the easy-to-use ice pick, and Freeman's charismatic energy, a further cause of the great dam-burst of lobotomy was the award of the 1949 Nobel Prize for Medicine to Moniz for his pioneering work in psychosurgery. Freeman was acutely disappointed to go unrewarded himself, but was at least pleased that he was invited to nominate Moniz for the prize.

Moniz's award sealed the future of tens of thousands of psychiatric patients, for it squashed many of the existing reservations about the operation, and more people were lobotomized in the three years after he received the prize than in the previous fourteen years. Nearly twice as many women as men were lobotomized. Freeman was very busy, and began to get quite fussy; he wanted to operate on patients within two years of their being institutionalized, and, in the case of schizophrenics, within the first year of illness. Quite simply, getting them earlier made the operation's results look better. Over 70 per cent of those admitted to institutions recovered anyway, and if they had been lobotomized early on, it was impossible to tell whether it was due to, or in spite of, the operation. Freeman would proudly say it was the former. He hated operating on chronic, hopeless cases; they were OK to practice on, but they made his recovery statistics look bad. First sold as an operation to be used as a last resort, the lobotomy had now become the first step to creating a manageable personality. Even problem children were being lobotomized. If everybody had their frontal lobes snipped at birth, there'd be an end to sorrow in the world. By 1950, in his frenzy of activity, Freeman had crossed and recrossed America eleven times on what he called his 'head-hunting' expeditions, promoting the ice pick, looking for new patients, checking up on his old ones. He found a partner, Dr Jonathan Williams, to replace the departed Watts. Williams was often shocked at Freeman's cavalier use of the ice pick, wielded anywhere at any time, but for Freeman, the passionate prophet of psychosurgery, these were his golden years.

By the early 1950s reservations about the effects of the lobotomy could be heard. Its use as a first, rather than a last resort, by amateur surgeons who did not even bother to give the patient a preliminary psychiatric report, was rife. Post-operative infections and simple fatalities were common; autopsies showed that large areas of brains, not selected nerves, were utterly destroyed. Astonishingly, there had still been no reliable sustained studies of the effects on patients, only Freeman's eternally optimistic data. Though some patients did continue to pursue their professional and private lives after the operation, it was impossible to state that this was because of the surgery. It was, furthermore, impossible to judge 'recovery' in many; they were often so different. The inert, emotionless, inhuman quality of many lobotomized, who were everywhere to be seen, began to revolt the public, though thousands still submitted relatives for the operation. As early as 1951, even the Soviet Union, where psychiatric abuse was rife, had stopped performing the lobotomy on ideological grounds: it produced unresponsive people who were fixed and unchangeable.

Lobotomy was suddenly seen for what it was: not a cure, but a way of managing the patient. It was just another form of restraint, a mental strait-jacket nailed permanently over the brain. It did not create new people; it subtracted from the old ones. It was an act of defeat, of frustration.

The Director of the New York State Psychiatric Institute, Nolan Lewis, asked: 'Is quieting a patient a cure? Perhaps all it accomplishes is to make things more convenient for those who have to nurse them ... the patients become rather childlike ... they are as dull as blazes. It disturbs me to see the number of zombies that these operations turn out ... it should be stopped.'

In 1952 chlorpromazine, the first of the new generation of revolutionary tranquillizers for schizophrenia, and depression, was tested in France. It signalled the end for Walter Freeman. From now on, he would be 'the ice pick lobotomist', with a rapidly diminishing clientele and shrinking reputation.

By 1954, everybody was on drugs; psychopharmacology had hit America, and the manufacturers of the biggest-selling tranquillizer, Thorazine, could literally not make enough to slake popular thirst for the chemical. Most neurosurgeons and psychiatrists who had practiced lobotomy tossed away their instruments with relief.

Not so Freeman; he took to the road, 'head-hunting' again, visiting the fifty-five hospitals in the twenty-three states where he had once gloriously wielded his ice pick on hundreds of people. He was obsessed with producing a follow-up study that would justify his work. He firmly believed that the pendulum would swing his way again, but by the end of the 1950s he was performing only a trickle of operations. His name had become tarnished; he found it hard to get on the staff of hospitals, and colleagues referred few patients to him.

At the 1960 World Psychiatry Congress, Freeman presented the results of his follow-up studies, claiming they showed that 85 per cent of his private trans-orbital patients were now at home, and two-thirds of them were 'usefully occupied'. His data were so anecdotal, so subjective, that they were not taken seriously. At the same time, a ten-year study on British patients was released which did not make such encouraging reading. Then, in 1962, *One Flew Over the Cuckoo's Nest* by Ken Kesey was published. The Pulitzer-Prize-winning novel became a classic bestseller; it was a damning portrayal of a psychiatric hospital, and of the effects of lobotomy. It was all over for the psychosurgeons. Freeman was then sixty-seven years old; most would have had enough. Yet throughout his final years, he remained active, busying himself with projects including his memoirs, and the book on the tendency of introverted psychoanalysts to kill themselves. With typical aggression, he tried to add to the list the psychiatrist Harry Sullivan who had died in 1949. Freeman tried to prove he had killed himself. Sullivan had been a bitter opponent of lobotomy in general and Freeman in particular.

He also continued to tour the country in a specially equipped camper van, which he called his 'lobotomobile', visiting former patients and gathering 'evidence' of their recovery, determined to prove that his love of the blade and the ice pick had not been misguided.

In February 1967, he used his ice pick for the last time. The patient was actually one of the original ten on whom he had first tried the trans-orbital in secret, in his office in 1946. This was the third time he had administered an ice pick lobotomy to this woman; he had also done it in 1956. He made the customary deep frontal entry with his ice pick, but this time the old magic failed; he tore a blood vessel in the brain. She died within hours. Freeman had his surgical privileges removed.

He refused to see himself as defeated. He had by now lost two of his sons, and his wife would precede him to the grave. He treated his emotions with his habitual long walks, and, when told that he had diabetes, eliminated sugar from his diet, and cured himself. On May 1972, after a brief battle with cancer, he died, aged seventy-seven.

No one now remembers the drill, the leucotome, and the ice pick with any sentiment other than sadness and remorse. There is no doubt that Freeman believed in the integrity of his methods and motives, but he is now seen as a principal architect of tragedy, not hope.

Hydrotherapy

Hydrotherapy is one of the oldest means of treating insanity. It had no curative effect, and was used to 'quiet' lunatics. It was widely advocated in Germany in the late nineteenth century to treat psychiatric patients. The patient was placed in a large tub of water at a temperature somewhere between 98 and 102 degrees. A tarpaulin was stretched over the bath, allowing only the patient's head to protrude. The warm bath causes the skin to engorge with blood, which lowers the breathing rate, the pulse, and the blood pressure. Relaxation, and drowsiness followed. The patient might be left in this way for hours, or days. Baths were still being used well into this century, as were douches, wet packs, steam, spritzers, and hoses. The physician John H. Kellogg proposed the use of an extraordinary device: a combined rain-douche, horizontal jet, and multiple douche for 'neurasthenia and other disorders'. The German authorities even suggested that certain seas had different therapeutic powers: 'The calm waters of the Baltic are preferable for delicate, nervous constitutions, and the North Sea, with its stronger billows, may be recommended for torpid constitutions.'

* * * * *

Asylum conditions

In York Asylum, a cell measuring twelve feet by seven feet was found to contain thirteen incontinent women. At a madhouse in Bethnal Green, a woman subject to violent seizure was flung, hands and feet bound, into a pigsty; when she recovered, she was bound to a bed, and only allowed to walk with an iron bar linking her legs together. To this her hands were also chained. At Bethlehem in London, naked patients were kept in conditions resembling 'a dog kennel', and a man named **William Norris** was found to have been chained by his neck to a stone for nine years. Madwomen were chained by the ankles to the wall of a long gallery, their only clothes a single, filthy, homespun dress. Samuel Tuke, who in the early nineteenth century wrote the influential *Report on the Condition of the Indigent Insane*, gives the details of a complicated system employed at Bethlehem to control a reputedly dangerous madman. He was attached by a long chain that ran over the wall and thus permitted the attendant to lead him about without having to go within any distance of him. Around this man's neck was an iron ring, attached by a short length of chain to another ring which was allowed to slide the length of a vertical iron bar running from the floor to the ceiling of his cell. Thus, the inmate could lay, or crouch, or squat, or walk in a circle round the bar as his master at the end of the leash dictated. When reforms were finally instituted at Bethlehem, a man was found who had lived in a cell in this fashion for twelve whole years.

* * * * *

Continental asylums

On the European continent, madhouses had been quite as appalling as in Britain. In his *Report on the Care of the Insane*, Desportes describes the cells of La Salpêtrière at the end of the eighteenth century as 'miserable and often fatal,' because, 'in winter, when the Seine rose, those cells situated at the level of the sewers became not only more unhealthy, but worse still, a refuge for a swarm of huge rats, which during the night attacked the unfortunates confined there, and bit wherever they could reach them; madwomen have been found with feet, hands and faces torn by bites.' Goguel said of the same prison that there were 'madwomen ... chained like dogs at their cell doors, and separated from keepers, by a long corridor protected by an iron grille; through this grille is passed their food and the straw on which they sleep; by means of rakes part of the filth that surrounds them is cleaned out.' At Strasbourg, another French inspector found a kind of human stable: 'For troublesome madmen, and those who dirtied themselves, a kind of cage, or wooden closet which could at the most contain one man of middle height have been devised.' These cages had gratings, not floors, and were raised above the ground, so that one would not have to let the man out of the cage in order to clean it. He had a little straw thrown across the grating inside the cage; when this was covered in excrement or the remains of food, it dropped through.

* * * * *

Different approaches to early brain surgery

Watts and Freeman were very different personalities. Watts was a relaxed man, who by his own admission was inclined to 'make things simple'. Freeman liked drama. Their differing temperaments were illustrated in their attitudes towards obtaining cerebro-spinal fluid from patients for testing purposes. Watts used the orthodox lumbar puncture, which was in itself a painful and potentially lethal process in which the patient was strapped down before fluid was extracted by syringe from the lumbar region. Freeman developed a rapid, violent and highly dangerous method which got his adrenalin going. It was quite shocking to watch. He simply made the patient straddle a chair, fold their arms over the back and drop their head forward. Then, holding their head in one hand, Freeman used the other to drive a hypodermic needle into the top of the neck, through the gap at the base of the skull-bone, and into the cistern magna where the spinal fluid gathers. A millimetre out, either way, and he would pierce the brain-stem, killing the patient. He loved to perform this operation in front of people. He called it his 'Jiffy' spinal tap.

* * * * *

Lobotomy

By 1938, a number of neurosurgeons throughout America were tentatively experimenting with lobotomy. One major reservation that many had to the operation was that they could not see what they were doing. In Jacksonville, Florida, a surgeon named J.G.Lyerly attempted to correct what he called this lack of 'prudent visibility' during the operation, and developed the 'open' method of lobotomy. In this a large section of the patient's skull over the frontal lobes was removed, like taking the cover off a fuse box. The lobes were lifted or pushed aside to allow direct access to the white matter beneath, and the surgeon then, by the light of a little torch, used a knife to cut the fibres and an electrical device to 'coagulate' the nerves, which crackled, hissed, and popped gruesomely as the tissue was seared, like a soldering iron at work. It really was quite a large-scale business, and the surgeon looked somewhat like a mechanic bending over the engine of a car, trailing a number of complex surgical tools. Watts said disparagingly of this method: 'The surgeon sees what he cuts but does not know what he sees,' and added ominously: 'It is easy to get lost in the frontal lobes.' Lyerly's method was important in allaying natural fears among psychiatrists that stemmed from a general ignorance of the layout of the brain. After one presentation of his work, a psychiatrist, who had previously had his doubts about lobotomy, said that he would instantly write to the 'relatives and friends of his patients,' and 'see if I can possibly induce them to take this chance.'

* * * * *

James Poppen's 'superior approach' lobotomy

An 'open-topped' form of lobotomy was developed by James Poppen, a Boston neurosurgeon. Even Freeman described it as 'gross', though perhaps there was a touch of professional spleen in his remark. Poppen made very large holes in the top of the head, and then used electrical and suction devices to fry, and then suck up the brain fibres. Freeman compared the technique to 'dipping a vacuum cleaner into a bucket full of spaghetti,' and said the effects on the brain were 'horrifying'. Watts was far more circumspect, and implicitly acknowledged the element of rivalry that was growing among neurosurgeons, and to which Freeman was particularly sensitive. 'We claimed our method was the best,' said Watts, 'but it's hard to know.'

* * * * *

Egas Moniz and the leucotome

Moniz knew that alcohol was liable to cause considerable, peripheral damage with unknown effects. He had actually designed and ordered a special cutting instrument with which to perform this operation and the many others he anticipated. It was called a leucotome, and was being manufactured in Paris. 'Leukos' is Greek for 'white' and the name of this instrument translates as 'white-matter knife'. It was to be an ingeniously simple device, modelled on the humble apple-corer. Indeed, it was not the last device used in psychosurgery to be inspired by the contents of the kitchen drawer.

The leucotome was a long, slender, tubular steel shaft, with a plunger at one end. When the shaft had been inserted into the brain, the plunger was depressed. In response, at the other end, sunk into the white matter, a thin looped piece of stainless steel wire popped out. The operator would then simply rotate the device, and the loop of wire would cut out a core of brain tissue. The plunger was pulled up, the loop retracted, and the leucotome could then be withdrawn. The little, lost islands of the mind detached in this way would simply float around until they dissolved. Unfortunately, the leucotome was not yet ready, and Moniz was impatient, so alcohol sufficed.

Lop' em, chop' em, shock' em

Civilization is confounded in the face of madness. This confusion has set in train a series of ever-escalating responses. In this century increasingly drastic, and, to our minds, cruel forms of intervention have been practiced: the removal of internal glands, gassing with carbon dioxide, shock therapy with the fear drug metrazol, and insulin-coma therapy progressing, inevitably, to the desperate act of lobotomy.

The journey towards the knife, the drill, the apple-corer and the ice pick begins with the division between body and mind that man sensed within himself. Five hundred years before the birth of Christ, Hippocrates, the Greek physician and patron of the modern medical arts, declared the brain to be the source of intellect, and the heart the organ of emotions.

Theories of lunacy
Galen, the anatomist, whose theory of four 'humours' that ruled man – blood, phlegm, choler, and black bile – was to predominate in medical thought and philosophy alike, was the natural successor to Hippocrates, believing that the heart was a warm, red space, and therefore more likely to be the origin of emotions, whereas the brain was cold and grey, and the obvious home of the rational intellect. In Galen's system, the four types of humours listed above corresponded to four types of character: sanguine, phlegmatic, choleric, and melancholic. Madness arose from an imbalance among the four humours leading to over-accentuated versions of the four characters. Hence madness was an affliction of the body, and could be treated by purging, bleeding, and other forms of simple (and ineffective) treatment.

Ranged against the Galenist was the Aristotelian tradition of thought. In this, madness has a specific link with the mind. It may even be indicative of exceptional, visionary qualities. Aristotle is alleged to have asked why all those eminent in politics, sciences, and the arts 'suffer from black bile?'

In 1621, the English writer Robert Burton published his extraordinary *Anatomy of Melancholy,* a collection of musings on the mysteries of madness. Melancholy had a myriad forms, but all were equally engaging, and Burton saw melancholy as a sign of mental individuality; its sufferers were 'of a deep reach, excellent apprehension, judicious, witty and wise'.

This essential divide in thinking, between those who saw madness as an organic illness, and those who saw it as a condition of the mind to be treated psychologically, was to persist among physicians of the modern era; the neurologists would be of the former opinion, the psychiatrists of the latter.

Spleen or the 'English disease'

During the eighteenth century, the notion of 'melancholy' was supplanted by that of 'spleen'. Spleen was taken to refer to a whole host of then fashionable mental conditions, vapours, hypochondriasis, hysteria, and also that organ of the same name, which Galen had supposed to be the source of his 'black bile'. Spleen tended to be an affliction of the rising middle class. It was, as many physicians of the time remarked, difficult to treat as it tended to mimic other illnesses. Overseas, it was known as 'the English malady', and blamed on England's climate, diet, and sedentary life enjoyed by its wealthy inhabitants. Many intellectuals were delighted to be informed they were suffering from mild insanity.

Spleen was perceived to be different from common madness;

its arrival marked a sharp divergence in the way other forms of insanity were treated. There had always been madness among the poor, in the shape of lunatics, but it was largely ignored, the lunatics contained within their village communities, or shipped out of the way and kept moving from town to town. Still, throughout the Middle Ages the fool had his place in the scheme of things, and was thought to be endowed with peculiar religious significance, and insight. In the eighteenth century, with the advent of the 'age of reason' attitudes changed; common madness became a social embarrassment which had to be shut away.

Public madhouses

In England, an Act of 1714 attempted to distinguish lunatics from other vagrants and empowered the local authorities to detain them in madhouses at the expense of the local parish. For over a hundred years, until the creation of the huge Victorian county asylums in the mid-nineteenth century, private madhouses, which took in the lunatics for easy money, flourished.

In theory, at this time, madness was perceived as an exclusively mental problem, the consequence of a losing battle fought between reason and imagination, an imbalance between man's rational and sensitive souls, and a variety of decadence. It could only be conquered in an intellectual way, though this might require the adoption of a stringent routine. Madness indicated some defect in reasoning; so the will needed to be trained to deal with this. In practice, for the confined, lunatic poor, no treatment was administered, simply restraint, and appalling abuses were rampant.

Not the least of these was the use of madness as an entertainment. It was an old custom in the Middle Ages to display the insane as an object of curiosity. When madmen began to be incarcerated as a matter of course, the custom did not disappear, but rather grew. It was as if the madhouse, in which insanity was now concentrated, had the resources of a theatre.

As late as 1815, the Bethlehem madhouse exhibited lunatics every Sunday, admission one penny. The annual revenue from these visits amounted to £400, which amounts to an astonishing 96,000 admissions a year. In France, the madmen at the Bicêtre hospital provided traditional entertainment for the middle classes, and the attendants used whips to make the mad perform their dances. At the asylum of Charenton, the director, Coulmier, actually organized theatrical performances, in which the inmates were sometimes actors, sometimes spectators, and over which the Marquis de Sade, incarcerated for his sexual vices, famously presided. One observer wrote that 'the insane who attend these theatricals were the object of the attention and curiosity of a frivolous, irresponsible, and often vicious public. The bizarre attitudes of these unfortunates and their condition provoked the mocking laughter, and the insulting pity of the spectators.' Madness was goaded into pure spectacle. Towards the end of the nineteenth century, as a concession, only the mad were allowed to exhibit themselves, and each other.

County asylums

The madness of King George III, a series of shocking public reports on the conditions of private madhouses, and a conviction, in an age of growing scientific confidence and social philanthropy, that the poor and insane would respond to the rational treatment advocated previously for the wealthy, spurred the creation of county asylums. When they finally opened, they were intended to cure with enlightened 'moral therapy'; they were not to restrain their inmates, but to provide a round of education, therapeutic work, and simple treatments such as showers and baths.

To the Victorians' dismay, the population of the insane rapidly expanded to overwhelm the asylums; they were so engulfed that treatment of any sort was no longer possible, only control and restraint. Though asylums were still bewildered by the symptoms of madness, the problems they faced were at root largely social: 75 per cent of those committed to asylums were simply paupers incarcerated under the Poor Law, the majority of them women, whose poverty and consequent insanity, where it existed, was the result of a rapidly changing economic climate which had caused the disintegration of their communities, families, and individual functions. For many women it was better inside than out, and they retreated into mental disorder. During the latter half of the nineteenth century, the number of wealthy patients at private clinics increased by 100 per cent; the number of pauper lunatics rose by nearly 400 per cent. Madness was now a social epidemic, a terrible problem without solution.

Lacking the ability to address the socio-economic factors that were turning the whole newly industrialized world crazy, physicians were further prevented from tackling this crisis by a lack of a coherent classification of mental disorders.

Given impetus by pathological anatomy (the examination of cadavers), the objective classification of physical diseases was proceeding apace. By peering into dead bodies, sickness was linked with diseased organs and their particular, impaired functions. By contrast, the classification of mental disorders was still largely a matter of opinion and observation of exterior behaviour. Things had changed little since, in 1604, Sir Edward Coke had designated four categories of madness: the idiot or fool natural; he who had once been of good and sound memory and 'by the visitation of God had lost it'; the lunatic who enjoys lucid intervals; and he who has rendered himself mad by his own act as a drunkard. In 1798, Philippe Pinel, the French physician, identified another four groups: mania, melancholia, dementia, and idiocy, but admitted that this was as far as medical knowledge stretched.

Even with the opportunities afforded by the study of anatomy, mental disorders remained an insoluble mystery. In looking for the diseased organs which were responsible, should one look in the body or the brain?

Somatic solutions

Although, for the meantime, this search was unproductive, a great deal of theory flourished. A growing body of physicians, rebelling against the fruitless work of psychiatrists in the asylums, were seeking what are called somatic or organic solutions to the problems of mental illness: that is, physical cures. They anticipated the eventual discovery that mental disorder had physical roots. Vague mental disorders would then become mental diseases. Once these had been called by their proper names, and the airy behavioural tags the psychiatrists gave them were discarded, the mystery of madness would melt away, as would the social crisis. The physicians who pursued this goal became neurologists, those concerned with the diagnosis and treatment of diseases of the nervous system.

While waiting for the 'mental diseases' to be discovered, neurologists resorted to various nonsensical forms of pseudo-diagnostic terminology. Patients were suffering from 'nervous prostration', 'nervous disintegration', 'cerebral neurosis', and 'neurasthenia'.

Mental disorders in women

Mental disorders of women were of great interest for the Victorians, providing much opportunity for specious diagnosis. Every doctor and gynaecologist also fancied himself as a neurologist when it came to the female, and hundreds of specialists in 'hysteria', and 'neurasthenia' sprang up. Their clientele was boosted by the apparent rise in female insanity. As the asylum statistics show, women accounted for the majority of admissions; many of these were unemployed, or former servants, which led the Victorians to speculate that there must be somewhere a particular mental disease that only struck at nannies. The disease was, of course, low income. Even for middle-class women who were not driven there by poverty, the single-sex asylum, where the day was spent in mild exercise, reading and sewing, often offered a more interesting, and gentler environment than Victorian home life. The Victorians, who thought of little else but sex, were obsessed with repressing sexuality, and Victorian textbooks offered exclusively sexual reasons for female insanity. It was due to the uterus, the menstrual cycle, and the menopause. Women were simply subject to so much change; how could they be inherently sane? Women were constantly monitored for the faintest fluctuation in mood, for unsubmissive behaviours, or for unnatural urges, such as making sexual demands of their husbands (John Ruskin was delighted to dump his wife into an asylum for this very reason) and were summarily diagnosed as suffering from 'mania', or 'melancholia'.

The gynaecologist, surgeon, and self-styled neurologist Isaac

Baker-Brown was not alone in blaming it all on the clitoris; few, however, have acted so decisively on their beliefs.

Using his little scissors ('I always prefer the scissors,' he wrote) Baker-Brown snipped the clitoris off scores of women. His catch-all remedy for female 'madness' was this clitoridectomy, which he performed, principally against their will, on the wives and daughters of respectable Victorians, some of whom had done little more than indulge in the aberration of 'serious reading'.

Baker-Brown's little volume *On the Curability of Certain Forms of Insanity,* published in 1866, is a classic of medical literature: assured, self-important, deeply misogynist, and risible if it were not so horrible. In the introduction he announces that the greatest 'mischief' in the nervous centre is caused by 'peripheral excitement' – his euphemism for masturbation, for it was not just the clitoris, but what women did with it, that distressed him. Sadly he observes: 'Daily experience convinces me that all unprejudiced men must adopt, more or less, the practice which I have thus carved out.'

Baker-Brown linked all female psychological ills to the 'pudic nerve': they were not mental problems, but 'physical illnesses amenable to medical and surgical treatment' which 'common charity' demanded he dealt with swiftly, and thereby remake these unfortunate women into 'happy and useful members of society'. He defends himself against objections to his trade with a self-righteousness that would be familiar to later ears: ' I can hardly conceive how such a question can be raised against a method of treatment which has for its object the cure of a disease.'

Baker-Brown listed eight ascendant degrees of female madness caused by 'peripheral excitement': hysteria, spinal irritation, epileptoid fits, cataleptic fits, epileptic fits, idiocy, mania, and death. These seem to have been interchangeable as he saw fit. As evidence that female masturbation led to death, Baker-Brown cited the case of a girl aged nineteen, 'who had for many years been in a metropolitan hospital suffering from acute headaches... for two years she had been perfectly blind ... was found dead, with every evidence of having expired during a paroxysm of excitement.'

A thirty-two-year-old whom her husband said was subject to violent fits in which she flew at him was subjected to the 'usual operation', after which the surgeon was pleased to note that she became a 'good wife'. A young woman of twenty, whose vagina and clitoris had already been the target of caustic fluids, was diagnosed as suffering from 'spinal irritation' caused by the usual vice, which was strongly denied, as her guardian claimed she was 'very religious'. Baker-Brown snipped her anyway. Another woman of the same age, who 'would not marry', and who indulged in 'serious reading', and was 'disobedient to her mother' was clearly a case of 'mental delusion'; same problem, same solution. A married woman aged thirty, who after having three children in rapid succession grew to hate her husband, was faced with Baker-Brown as the only alternative to a divorce which would have ruined her. She was put to the knife, having been diagnosed as suffering from 'incipient mania'. Afterwards, the surgeon matchmaker was happy to see that she had become a 'happy and healthy wife and mother', which led him to muse on the marriages his operation might save: 'If medical and surgical treatment were brought to bear, all such unhappy measures such as divorce would be obviated.' A spinster aged thirty-four, who had 'never had an offer of marriage' and who was thought peculiar because she went for long walks in the country, read furiously, and said 'people's faces were masks' was diagnosed insane by Baker-Brown and had her clitoris removed. She was fortunate to get away with that, because by now, Baker-Brown had got bored with merely removing the clitoris and had started excising the whole labia.

Baker-Brown's theories can be seen in one shape or another, popping up recurrently in the history of psychiatric treatment: the origin of what the age terms 'insanity' is traced to one organ, which can be lopped off, or chopped out. It is a question of finding which organ one believes the deviant personality to be located in. Then, it was the sexual organs, because masturbation was regarded with such horror, particularly in women, who were thereby achieving an illicit independence. Later, it would be the frontal lobes of the brain.

The rift between psychology and neurology
On a more mundane level, it was at this point, in the nineteenth century, that the great rift between psychiatrists and neurologists began: the professional rivalry, and the battle to find the roots of insanity. Both groups were fighting to establish themselves as rightful rulers of the kingdom of the insane, and were to argue bitterly over territory. Their conflict would help pave the way to the lobotomy. The battleground was America.

The situation was, in reality, utterly confused. Psychiatry, which had control over the burgeoning American asylums, was dominated by the 'moral therapists', for whom cures were still connected with teaching self-discipline. They eschewed drugs and advocated exercise, gentle work, and education. Unfortunately, half the patients psychiatrists were treating were suffering from conditions that we would recognize as having organic origins: syphilis, atherosclerosis, and alcohol poisoning. Asylums, as in Britain, had little time to treat, and fell back on various forms of restraint: guards, bars, chairs with straps, and the camisole or straitjacket. Conversely, neurologists, armed with their reflex hammers, their tuning forks, and their ophthalmoscopes for peering into the eyes and their pins which were stuck in to test for sensation, kept trying to tell people whose complaints were entirely psychological that they had a disease.

The neurologists took heart from the work of two people, Gall and Alzheimer. Gall was an early nineteenth-century anatomist and phrenologist – one who studied the bumps on the head and linked them to specific aspects of the human personality. Some of his anatomical work on the brain was constructive; much of his phrenology was risible. Gall showed that some method was possible for neurologists; and feeling the bumps on people's heads gave them something to do with their hands.

Alois Alzheimer

In 1904 Alois Alzheimer discovered that one form of premature dementia was linked to 'senile plaques' in the brain. Here, at last, was a mental disease, to which he gave his name, gleefully noting that there would undoubtedly be more so-called 'psychiatric disease' for which physical causes could be found.

At the same time, around the turn of the century, the work of various physicians began to reveal the enormous extent to which syphilis was responsible for 'general paresis', also known as 'general paralysis of the insane', 'general paralysis', and 'dementia paralytica'. In its terrifying final stages it literally caused paralysis as well as severe mental disintegration and death.

Paresis had long been claimed by psychiatrists to be caused by intemperance and immorality. It was a product of visualization with its demands on 'physical and mental powers, competition, reckless and feverish pursuit of wealth and social position, overstudy, overwork, unhygienic modes of life, the massing of people in large cities, the indulgence in tea, coffee, tobacco, stimulants, and social and sexual excesses, and artificial modes of life,' wrote T. H. Kellogg in 1897. Psychiatrists had ignored the fact that paresis was frequently hereditary, because it was in reality hereditary syphilis. Now this prince of mental disorders was found to be a disease, which left the neurologists and psychiatrists squabbling over who should treat it. Paresis was a central element in psychiatric theory, and they were reluctant to relinquish it without a fight.

Soon, the neurologists said, all mental disorders would be found to have their points of 'somatic' origin. They sneered at the emergent practice of psychoanalysis instigated by Freud, himself a former neurologist who was profoundly disappointed by the split between the organic theories of the neurologists and the equally passionate non-organic beliefs of psychiatrists. He wanted a theory that reunited the body and the mind, that connected mental illness and physical illness.

Dr Charles Burr, President of the American Neurological Association, told his members that 'Freud had a dirty mind', and that was the end of the matter. While a young man Walter Freeman, later the champion of the lobotomy, tried his hand at a session of psychoanalysis with a woman who claimed she suffered from extreme anal irritation. Freeman regarded her complaint as psychosomatic, and imaginary; she was later found to have a very real, large, and hideously painful anal fissure, which convinced Freeman he was right to hereafter avoid such claptrap.

For psychiatrists the 'talking cure' was too complex, and time-consuming for them to practice in the frantic and hopeless atmosphere of asylums. It remained a treatment for the wealthy.

No convincing theory of mental disorder appeared; no more organic causes were discovered; the populations of the asylums continued to increase, particularly in the wake of the First World War. Although more rigorous approaches to diagnosing and classifying mental disorders were developed, the textbooks remained rather short of suggested cures.

In the absence of any certain cures, a positively wild spirit of *laissez-faire* prevailed. Virtually any exotic and desperate treatment was now tried, provided it had the potential to treat large numbers of patients with a minimum of trained staff. This made the somatic treatments advocated by the neurologists particularly attractive. In any case, psychiatrists were by 1920 so baffled and helpless in the face of the vast population of inmates that they were secretly prepared to try anything Although they quarrelled about theory publicly, in practice there had for some time been little difference in the way psychiatrists and neurologists treated their patients. A psychiatrist who publicly defended a psychological approach to mental disorders frequently prescribed the primitive sedatives opium, or barbiturates, or the lifestyle changes that neurologists used. When prescribing their 'rest cures', neurologists would hastily deny that these had anything to do with 'mind cures', but were intended to build up the body's resources.

Surreptitiously, without public or personal acknowledgement, the two opposed sides were merging in the need for a violent, and despairing assault on the human psyche. The treatments essayed became more and more outlandish.

Sleep therapy

Sleep therapy or 'prolonged narcosis' was widely used from 1920 onwards, though its application can be traced back as far as the 1870s. The rationale for this treatment was that mental disorder was the product of an exhausted nervous system which a prolonged sleep would restore to a normal state. By means of barbiturates and opium, mental patients were kept in a comatose sleep for periods of between one and two weeks; in some instances for as long as a month. While heavily drugged, they were allowed to surface briefly from their deathly slumbers in order to eat and defecate. As with all the following treatments, enormous successes were claimed for narcosis, though these were never proved. The beneficial effects were attributed, in the hopeful terminology of the time, to such vague causes as 'improved cellular oxidation', 'healing of brain inflammation', or the establishment of a balance between 'the brain's inhibitory and excitatory forces'. The treatment was still used in the 1960s in the Soviet Union (a dubious indicator of validity), where doctors induced spleen with electric shocks. In the 1970s the Australian Dr Harry Bailey was still busily practicing 'deep-sleep therapy', inducing near coma-like states in psychiatric patients suffering in many cases from mild depression. During the course of the sleep they were subjected to systematic shock treatment. Many never woke up; some woke up years later. Bailey himself was later pronounced insane.

Other bizarre treatments

A professor at the University of Wisconsin, Arthur Solomon Loevenhart, tried 'cerebral stimulation', injecting schizophrenics with sodium cyanide, which he claimed was marginally successful. Then, in another attempt to excite the nervous system, he and his colleagues ordered patients to breathe in a gas mixture containing 30 per cent carbon dioxide, which was 3,000 times greater than the percentage then found in the atmosphere. Dizzy and hyped-up by the gas, patients appeared to react positively, leading Loevenhart to claim that they had achieved 'cerebral stimulation' in 'dementia praecox, manic depressive insanity, and involutional melancholia'. The shock treatment, after which long-catatonic patients apparently woke up and talked, aroused great interest, and soon everybody was gassing their local lunatics with some rough admixture of carbon dioxide. Psychoanalysts even found a way to explain its success as the 'consequence of awakening unconscious fears which were then assimilated into conscious thought.' After Loevenhart's death, his disciples moved on to drugs, using the 'truth drug' (sodium amytal) on schizophrenics, as a way of probing those repressed corners of the human mind.

Henry Cotton

One of the most prominent figures in this era of bizarre treatments was Henry Cotton, progenitor of the most generalized somatic therapy of the whole strange selection. Medical Director of the New Jersey Hospital, and a former colleague of Alois Alzheimer, Cotton proposed that all mental disturbances were caused by toxic substances produced by bacteria at infectious sites throughout the body. In Cotton's system, all psychotic patients had infected teeth. Infections lurked even in those that appeared healthy to the untrained eye. 'Focus infection' could be eliminated only by extraction: if in doubt, yank it out. Tonsils were also a source of lurking insanity; best to take them out as young as possible. The gastro-intestinal system held all sorts of horrors, especially the stomach and colon. One could not completely remove the offending organs, but one could 're-section' the colon, that is, cut away part of it, an operation he prescribed for 250 individuals in the first year it was tried. That a third of the patients died was blamed on incompetent surgeons. In women, the cervix was found, Cotton reckoned, to be infected in about 80 per cent of mental patients. The source of infection was, logically, 'enucleated', with the core of the cervix removed, though in some cases things had got so bad that Cotton felt obliged to remove the fallopian tubes and ovaries to boot, and even the uterus. In men, it was found less necessary to excise infected seminal sacs, as men tended to be cleaner in that area. Men are generally squeamish about lopping off testicles.

When Cotton first publicly gave details of his work and his supporting battery of statistics, claiming phenomenal rates of success, he had already chopped out the teeth, intestines, and reproductive organs of 1,400 patients. In 1923, detailed studies carried out by other interested parties showed, to their disappointment, no discernible difference in rate of improvement between Cotton's patients and others who had rather more of their organs left. Pioneers of drastic therapy tended to be over-optimistic with their own data; generally there were a number of incidental deaths which required justifying.

Cotton's work had, in principle, the support of the great psychiatrist Adolf Meyer, who had even written an introduction for Cotton's book. Meyer was the most respected living individual in the field, and a man who embraced both somatic and psychological therapies in his 'psychobiological' approach to mental disorder. While committed at a far remove to biological interpretations of insanity, he stressed the importance of nursing, occupational therapy, and social work; sufferers were to be socialized. While he could discuss all other theories of the cause of insanity, he had no theory of insanity himself, and, while giving the impression of being immensely practical, prescribed no particular course of treatment other than 'common sense'; hence, in an uncertain realm, he was king of the undecided and much respected for it. A fine writer without saying anything original, he was a great comfort to the majority who, like him, cautiously welcomed each new treatment for fear of being proved wrong. Meyer's support gave considerable medical weight to several violent treatments, including lobotomy, which quite transgressed his boundaries of 'common sense'.

The public arguments provoked by Cotton's work at a lecture he gave were very similar to those aroused by the lobotomies of Freeman and Watts a few years later. Critics questioned the ethics of the casual fashion in which Cotton performed castration, colostomy, hysterectomy, and cholectomy; and they questioned his statistics, pointing out that most of the patients he claimed to have cured would have recovered anyway.

Others, as one would expect, praised Cotton for acting positively, for being an optimist, for projecting a public image of hope. Another audience member attacked the critics of Cotton for standing in the way of 'innovation'. 'We do not want to put ourselves in a position of opposition to anything that promises benefit or good to our patients,' he declared. 'We need to do more of the work Dr Cotton is doing.' Some had been trying

Cotton's techniques on their own patients, and reported success.

In 1933, ten years after studies had discredited Cotton's extravagant assertions, he was still widely respected, and wrote an article entitled *The Physical Causes of Mental Disorders* for the American *Mercury* magazine, in which he was described as one of the leading psychiatrists in the United States. The magazine was run by a man called Mencken, who held that 'so-called mental disease' was the result of physical disorders, and took particular pleasure in embarrassing psychiatrists with opposing views at every possible opportunity. In his article, Cotton reasserted his beliefs and stated that: 'We have estimated that 80 per cent of the so-called functional type of mental disorders are not only due to infected teeth and tonsils but also to congenital malformation of the colon, or large intestines. Relics of medical superstition and barbarism are being supplanted by up-to-date conceptions ... the inhuman neglect that has resulted from the old discredited philosophical dualism of mind and body is being overcome by the idea of a unified mind and body.'

The last part of this statement suggests that those who thought like Cotton could now confidently argue that their actions were creative and conciliatory. They had seized the moral high ground. Cotton was implying that those who believed the mind to be a separate entity from the body were the destructive forces, tearing the human in two. His drastic therapy was humane.

Electro-convulsive therapy

The stage was finally set for the lobotomy with the large-scale adoption of somatic shock treatments. These were, respectively, insulin-coma therapy, and metrazol-convulsion therapy, which were in wide use by 1935. Although electricity had long been used in surgery, electro-convulsive therapy was not initiated until 1938. These treatments were readily accepted because of the precedents for drastic treatment set by Cotton and Loevenhart, and they achieved great popularity among psychiatrists and neurologists alike, precisely because nobody could explain why they worked. They did not show that mental disorders were a physical disease, which pleased the psychiatrists, but they showed that medical intervention had an effect, which delighted the neurologists. The great divide between mind and body was bridged by avoiding the question. Anybody could administer these treatments without feeling they were deserting their principles.

The metrazol-convulsive treatment
Metrazol is also called cardiazol in Europe. It is a synthetic chemical, synonymous with fear. Injected into patients, it creates a 'metrazol storm' in the centre of the brain, and targets the more primitive parts of the mind with quite horrifying results. The patient experiences a level of primeval fear that is terrible to watch. Two American scientists experimenting with metrazol on humans were compelled to break with the tradition of objective scientific observation and note: 'One thing that has impressed us from the clinical perspective is the fleeting, but quite definite and almost animal-like expression of fear that appears just before the first convulsive tightening of the body... it is almost haunting in character and stays with the observer throughout the attack and afterwards ... it seems as if one is carried back in time ... to some primeval point.' Some researchers used metrazol on patients for three-hour periods.

The metrazol-convulsive treatment was the invention of a Hungarian, Joseph Ladislas von Meduna. From a conservative background, and with fascist sympathies, Meduna had an erratic medical education, periodically interrupted by stints of fighting in the First World War. While examining the brains of former epileptics and schizophrenics, Meduna came to believe that there were differences in the nerve cells between the two. From this (incorrect) observation he rapidly concluded that those subject to fits of an epileptic nature would not suffer from schizophrenia, and he decided to try to synthesize epilepsy in mental patients. He tried injecting several different chemicals to achieve the desired effect, and finally settled on camphor (a chemical relation of menthol), before switching to metrazol.

Meduna's work, for which he claimed about a 50 per cent success rate in treating previously inert schizophrenics, was quickly adopted for general usage, stimulated by Meduna's wide travels throughout Europe and the realization that shock treatment was more effective on common depressives than on schizophrenics. Meduna emigrated to America, and by 1940 every major mental institution in the country included on their menu a version of his metrazol-convulsive treatment.

Joseph Sakel and insulin coma therapy

Insulin coma was another traumatic form of therapy, and was again the pioneering work of an ambitious and forceful individual, in this case Joseph Sakel, a Viennese doctor of Polish-Jewish extraction. Working at the Lichterfelde Sanatorium in Berlin, which specialized in dealing with drug addicts and was particularly popular with the city's artistic community, Sakel accidentally gave an overdose of insulin to one of his patients, a morphine-addicted actress who was also receiving insulin for her diabetes.

The overdose of insulin lowered the glucose level in the actress's blood, depriving the brain of energy, and sent her into a mild coma. Sakel was highly concerned, but she recovered and found that her craving for morphine had subsided. Henceforth, he began to administer insulin overdoses to all the drug addicts, and in 1930 published a report on his work in which, without providing any supporting evidence, he claimed a 100 per cent success rate in curing morphine addiction.

Again by accident, he administered a serious overdose of insulin to a drug addict who also happened to be psychotic, precipitating a serious coma, after which Sakel said that the patient showed signs of mental improvement. Believing he had stumbled on something significant, Sakel began experimenting on animals in his own kitchen, and came to the conclusion that such deep and deathly comas could be safely controlled by a prompt injection of glucose. He moved quickly from theory to practice, and began inducing deep comas in schizophrenics. He relocated to Vienna, and continued his work, publishing a stream of papers in which he claimed a success rate of 88 per cent, which was frankly miraculous at a time when psychiatrists thought schizophrenia incurable.

Because patients did seem to show an immediate improvement, and because the therapy itself was so dramatically compelling and simple, it spread like wildfire. For American neurologists Sakel, like Alzheimer and Cotton, was a hero, and they celebrated the moral victory won over psychoanalysis and conventional psychiatrists who were now adopting *en masse* these organic methods of treatment. Foster Kennedy, Professor of Neurology at Cornell and Bellevue Hospital, wrote disparagingly, in the preface to the American edition of Sakel's work: 'In Vienna, at least one man had revolted from the obsession that only psychological remedies could benefit psychological ills ... we shall not again be content to minister to a mind diseased, merely by philosophy and words.'

Although he could not give a coherent explanation as to why it worked – indeed, his attempts to do so were acutely embarrassing and unnecessary, as the attraction of the treatment was that everybody could have their homespun theory – Sakel continued to publicize the virtues of insulin-coma therapy. His optimism clearly influenced the observation of others, for when several psychiatrists he had 'trained' in the technique were publicly asked how they had fared with their patients, they first said that they were a little disappointed with their results, which did not seem to be as good as Sakel's statistics had promised; but they hastened to make positive noises in as general a fashion as possible: 'All patients ... benefit to a greater or lesser extent,' said one, and another: 'There is not a shadow of a doubt in my mind that there has been a definite improvement in a number of cases.'

Extensive studies carried out through 1939–40 showed that, although the beneficial effects of insulin coma wore off quickly for the majority, there remained a slight improvement in a modest percentage of patients who had undergone the therapy. The degree of success was a fraction of that which Sakel had claimed. Interest in the procedure declined during the 1940s and it all but vanished with the introduction of modern drugs in the 1950s. Although it was still being occasionally advocated as an effective treatment for schizophrenia in the 1960s, it was utterly forgotten by the end of the decade.

Sakel was a tragic figure, a contradictory and difficult man whose lack of scientific grounding meant he could literally never speak the language. He responded with aggression and paranoia, later obsessively claiming himself to be the sole inventor of all shock therapies. A heart attack forced his early retirement in 1946. Alienated by his temperament from his former colleagues, he watched his treatment being discarded with bitterness. When he died in 1957 of another heart attack, alone and forgotten, only one medical journal carried an obituary.

It was in the context of these shock therapies that lobotomy was first practiced. One can see why it held such an appeal; like the shock treatments, it was a speculative business, and the practitioners could make up their own minds as to why they thought it worked. Practically, it was quicker and cheaper, requiring no hospitalization and little training or equipment; and it was, furthermore, dramatic, with rather uncanny overtones. Most importantly, perhaps, physicians had become accustomed to thinking only in terms of extreme measures in their conflict with mental disorder, and lobotomy appeared to be the correct response to desperate circumstances; it was what the public, as well as the physicians, wanted.

There is a familiar image in American films in which the two ends of the railroad, begun either side of the continent, meet in the desert. The workers gather round to watch the owner drive the last rivet in, joining so many opposites of culture, people, and climate. Lobotomy did this too; it united psychiatry and neurology, body and mind. But it was a misconceived gesture, for the rivet was a knife, and far from being the creative operation that it was said to be, the blade was turned, in a destructive act laden with frustration and anger, on that which refused to yield up its secrets: the mind of the patient.

Insulin shock therapy

By 1938, insulin shock therapy was being administered in 54 per cent of mental institutions, sometimes by itself, sometimes in combination with metrazol, and later with electric shock treatment. The press acclaimed it and encouraged popular belief in shock therapies as instant wonder cures, carelessly exaggerating Sakel's dubious statistics still further. The death rate for the treatment, which was not dwelt on, was a little over one in twenty in private hospitals and as much as three in twenty in public hospitals. Death occurred when a patient could not be retrieved from the coma. Non-fatal brain damage was more common, affecting about one in ten in private hospitals, and again, more in public institutions. That it was so popular is yet more bewildering when one considers how complex a business it had become, requiring a great deal of personal attention and care. Patients were kept in semi-darkness for six to ten weeks, given gradually escalating doses of insulin for five days of the week; they might be plunged into as many as fifty comas, which threw them into twitching, gasping and shouting convulsions. A shock-treatment ward was a scene from hell. A great number of trained nurses and doctors were required to supervise the grotesque process. Their task was not made easier by the lack of any standard procedure in the treatment; no one, least of all Sakel, knew what was actually happening to these people. The doctors just had to hope they were doing the right thing at the right time.

* * * * *

Electro-convulsive therapy

Electro-convulsive or electro-shock therapy was developed between the world wars by two Italians, Ugo Cerletti and Lucio Bini. While working, like Meduna, with epileptic patients Cerletti had become convinced that convulsions created some 'vitalizing' bodily secretion, which he and Bini tried to induce in animals by electric shocks. Unfortunately all the animals died. Then they realized that they should stop passing the current through the heart. They moved the electrodes to the head, with success, and in 1938 first tried their electro-convulsive therapy on a human. This was a lost schizophrenic, found wandering aimlessly around the train station in Rome, and obligingly supplied to the doctors by the police commissioner. They tried him at a low voltage without generating much of a twitch, so, ignoring his protests, they turned up the power. After acute spasms, he recovered, and was calm and talkative. Within a few years, electro-shock treatment was being used in half of America's mental institutions, and it gradually usurped both metrazol and insulin. Electro-shock therapy has remained a standard psychiatric treatment to this day, though it is now sparingly used. Again, although envisaged as a treatment for schizophrenia, it was found to be more effective on depressives; and, as with other shock treatments, no one understands how it works. Cerletti theorized that the 'vitalizing' secretion it created was something he called 'acro-amines', and thought that if he could find them in the blood of animals he had shocked, they could then be injected into humans. This would eliminate the need to induce convulsions which he did not think did any good in themselves and which he found unpleasant to watch. He never found his magical secretion.

* * * * *

Early skull-drillers

As neurologists and psychiatrists moved slowly towards direct physical intervention in the human brain, they looked for precedents. Apart from Gottlieb Burckhardt, mentioned elsewhere, a British surgeon called Claye Shaw had drilled holes in the skulls of patients at the Bamstead Asylum and penetrated the frontal lobes in an attempt to cure paresis, as had two American surgeons, Wagner and Fuller. An Estonian named Lodivicius Puusepp had attempted to treat mental patients by cutting the nerve tracts connecting the frontal lobes to the rest of the brain without much success. Later, in 1910, he drilled four or five holes in the heads of paresis victims and dropped a mixture of cyanide and mercury into the nerve connections. He said his treatment produced a 'notable improvement'.

* * * * *

Krafft-Ebbing's experiments

At the turn of the century, Richard von Krafft-Ebbing injected pus obtained from the sores of known syphilis victims into patients diagnosed by psychiatrists as suffering from 'general paralysis'. The guinea pigs did not develop syphilis, Krafft-Ebbing concluded, because they already had it. This completely unethical experiment was successful in showing that paresis had its roots in a disease. The first modern treatment for syphilis was the arsenic compound Salvarsan, Paul Ehrlich's 'magic bullet', the 606th chemical formula he had tried out. But neither it nor its immediate successors were successful in advanced cases of paresis. Then the psychiatrist Wagner-Jauregg arrived with his malaria shock treatment, for which he won the Nobel Prize in 1927. Wagner-Jauregg had started out by trying other fevers, tuberculosis, typhoid, and even erysipelas – having noticed that paresis patients were relieved in their suffering when treated with ointments that induced fever and lots of gooey pustules around the head. After the initial success of his malaria treatment, Wagner-Jauregg continued to use it, targeting those in the early stages of syphilis and claiming up to 80 per cent success. The malaria treatment was widely used in Europe and America, and when it became clear that it was fever, not malaria, that killed syphilis, a number of bizarre heat treatments evolved: hot baths, hot air, radiothermy, diathermy, infra-red light-bulb boxes and special sleeping bags were all used. After the First World War, it was alleged that Wagner-Jauregg's psychiatric clinic had used electric shock treatment to punish soldiers who were thought to be malingering, using powerful currents that resulted in death and suicide. Freud himself, a former classmate of Wagner-Jauregg's, was asked to lead an investigation. He cleared Wagner-Jauregg, but the stigma remained. Wagner-Jauregg was, and still is, the only psychiatrist to have been awarded the Nobel Prize for medicine. Consequently he and his dramatic therapies were the object of veneration and emulation by all neurologists and psychiatrists who believed in an organic, physical view of mental disorders. Among these was Walter Freeman.

The desire to pin down the source of madness to one or another organ manifested itself in the popular practice of removing the endocrine glands – those internal organs that produce vital secretions. Hence the ovaries, the testes, the adrenal, and the thyroid glands were removed from tens of thousands of mental patients throughout the world in the 1920s. It had long been suspected that hormonal imbalances caused fluctuations in mood, and created depression and irritability, and some neurosurgeons made a specific connection between 'mental disorders' in women, and their menstrual cycles, or the depression following pregnancy. Walter Freeman was interested in all this frenzied cutting going on around him, and conducted extensive autopsies on victims of depression in an attempt to find the effects of such surgery on the personality. He was disappointed. While there was, he thought, a connection between such general anomalies as already mentioned and the endocrine glands, he considered that excising them would have little effect on the actual personality.

Sigmund Freud and the talking cure

It seems likely, if the present trend of opinion is anything to go by, that at least some future historians of medicine will classify Freudian psychoanalysis as one of the most monumental medical blunders of all time. That comment is likely to infuriate large numbers of people who are devoted to Freud and all his works, but it is not made without adequate backing.

The Austrian psychiatrist Sigmund Freud (1856–1939) was not the originator, but was certainly the best-known guru of psychoanalysis. His ideas have had an immense influence on twentieth century culture. To some extent, this was because of his intense preoccupation with sexual matters at a time when such subjects were considered hardly suitable for polite society. This, of course, made them exceptionally interesting. In addition, the shocked rejection of his ideas made good advertising copy and, as a result, these ideas became widely known.

Freud was a man of extraordinary and powerful intellect, a precocious scholar who read Shakespeare at eight and steeped himself in the Latin, Greek, French and German classics. His early medical studies into neurology brought him into contact, in Paris, with the famous neurologist Jean Martin Charcot (1825–93), who had clearly recognised the influence of the mind on physical symptoms. Freud adopted Sir Francis Galton's method of free association, and, in the repressive times in which he lived, inevitably found a strong sexual content in the half-concealed thoughts of his patients. This so impressed him that he became convinced that sex was at the basis of everything, and he gradually evolved an empirical system of thought, based on literary rather than scientific principles. Freud repeatedly insisted that his methods were scientific and, although in the context of his time they may have been, they do not now appear to be so.

Freud concentrated on the unconscious mind and its actions as motivators of behaviour. He was deeply concerned with the role of sexual symbolism in thought and dreams, and came to regard every elongated object as symbolic of the penis and every receptacle as symbolizing the vagina. He believed, rightly, that early experiences have a profound effect on later behaviour and personality and that these experiences became repressed and lay hidden under layers of subsequent mental accretion, but could be uncovered by analysis. He asserted, without proof, that the uncovering of these early experiences would disperse the psychopathology which he claimed they had caused. As a result, millions of people have devoted a substantial proportion of their time (and money) to the analytic process, mostly with no discernible effect.

Freud's divisions of the mind

He proposed arbitrary divisions of the mind into ego, superego and id. He asserted that infants pass though three stages – oral (birth to 18 months), anal (two to five years) and phallic (five years onward), and that the personality could be fixed at any of these stages with dire consequences, curable only by psychoanalysis. He claimed that little boys want to kill their fathers and have sexual intercourse with their mothers – the Oedipus complex – and that they fear being found out and having their penises cut off – the castration complex. Later in his career he formulated the idea of the death wish – Thanatos – and used this to explain a good deal of the destructive elements in human behaviour. Throughout his life, he repeatedly modified his earlier ideas so that a detailed survey of his writings can be a little confusing.

Freud's publications aroused shock and horror, especially in the orthodox medical community. But they also brought him a degree of fame, not to say notoriety, which eventually was damaging to his judgement and led him to suppose that his assertions were infallible and that anyone who doubted them was wicked. Soon the Freudian school took on all the characteristics of a religion, including unquestioned dogma, an insistence on belief in spite of clear evidence to the contrary and the persecution of heretics. Two of the best-known defectors were Adler and Jung, each of whom formed his own schismatic school of psychological thought.

There is little in Freud's voluminous and widely-read literary output to support his assertion that he was a scientist in the sense we now understand the word. Most of his claims for psychoanalysis are essentially unverifiable but, even more damaging, are incapable of being disproved – a reliable feature, according to the philosopher Karl Popper (1902–94), of a pseudo-science. Adverse criticism is the lifeblood of real science, which is concerned with demonstrable and reliable knowledge. But Freud and his followers have always reacted aggressively to criticism, attributing the views of the critic to unresolved Oedipus complexes or other 'psychopathology'. The serious scientist, faced with this no-win situation, can only murmur that he or she would be ashamed to fall back on the *argumentum ad hominem* as a response to a criticism of one of his or her propositions. Scientific facts have nothing to do with the nature – other than their honesty – of the people who assert them.

Freud's major contribution to thought – and it is a very large one – was to draw attention to the powerful influence the unconscious mind has on behaviour and conscious thought. His school of psychoanalysis has been less successful and there is little or no evidence, apart from the assertions of its practitioners, that the application of Freudian ideas in psychoanalysis has any intrinsic value in the treatment of psychological disturbance. Close, one-to-one relations between humans can be highly therapeutic, especially if one of them is in a position of authority and purports to be keenly interested in the mental activities and problems of the other. But the outcome is more likely to depend on the experience, maturity and human and intellectual qualities of the dominant partner than on whether the 'patient' feared castration in infancy or was prevented from playing with his or her faeces.

Freudian psychoanalysis
Freudian psychoanalysis is based on a number of assertions which, in the minds of adherents, have become axioms. These are that:

- many important events in the mental life of the individual take place in the unconscious mind
- most of what goes on in the unconscious is concerned with sex and aggression
- these 'unconscious thoughts', 'wishes' and 'impulses' are a constant potential source of neurosis
- they are constantly being revealed by symbolism in dreams and by significant errors and puns ('Freudian slips'), which are often subtle expressions of sexual and aggressive impulses
- most of the troubles of mankind can, ultimately, be traced to little boys' repressed jealousy of their fathers' sexual access to their mothers (the Oedipus complex)

Freud claimed that the unconscious mind was accessible by a process of free association and that when repressed painful material was 'brought to the surface' and contemplated, the harm that it had been causing would be resolved. The analyst's function was a passive, detached, non-commenting and non-participatory guidance. This was the 'talking cure'. One might suppose that before putting forward, as scientifically valid, a method of treatment such as this, one should at least try it a considerable number of times. Freud's convictions, in this context, were in fact based on no more than a small handful of cases. The first of these was that of a twenty-one-year-old woman called Bertha Pappenheim, known, for reasons of privacy, as Anna O. This patient was introduced to Freud by a colleague called Josef Breuer. Freud had been trying hypnotism on his private patients with very little success. One day, Breuer told him that he had developed a talking treatment for hysteria and had used it successfully on Bertha. He had suggested to her that she should talk about anything that came into her head. After much indifferent chatter, the girl had come up with a story about her father's illness and death. This was recounted with a powerful emotional reaction and after that the symptoms she had been complaining of disappeared.

Both Breuer and Freud were deeply impressed by this incident and Freud interpreted it as a 'catharsis' – a Greek word for the effects of a purgative. His idea was that this repressed mischief was the cause of Bertha's trouble and now that it had been brought up and released, she was cured. Breuer got on so well with Bertha that his wife became jealous and he had the sense to stop seeing Bertha. Freud, however, continued to treat patients with the talking cure. Thus was psychoanalysis born. Unfortunately, Bertha's case notes turned up later in the

Bellevue Sanatorium in Kreutzlingen, Switzerland. These showed that Bertha's symptoms soon returned in full and that they were not due to hysteria, as Breuer and Freud had supposed, but to tubercular meningitis. Bertha's father had had a tubercular abscess in his chest and this had been opened and drained at home. In spite of this treatment, he had died.

In spite of Freud's claims about this case, it is now known that he was aware of at least some of the true facts of the matter. His disciple Jung, who also knew the facts, seems to have been more honest than his master and pointed out that the alleged cure had not been a cure at all. There is plenty of evidence that several of Freud's claimed cures were imaginary. A substantial literature exists proving that the facts of some of his cases were quite different from his accounts of them.

Even in Freud's lifetime, psychoanalysis quickly became a religion, with a systematised theology and a set of rigid dogmas. Minds were closed to other possibilities and heretics were persecuted. Evidence which supported the dogma was entertained; evidence against it was ignored. New prophets arose with ever more complex interpretations of the master's writings, and a vast exegetical literature was produced, much of which would try the credulity of anyone but a believer.

Whatever the merits of Freud's theories – and it has to be said that, wheat sifted from chaff, his contribution to thought was certainly important – the value of the application of them to the practical management of psychological disorder is now seen to be negligible. Significantly, Freud recognised, and taught, that unless a transference was achieved – that is unless the patient fell in love with, or otherwise became emotionally involved with, the analyst – psychoanalysis would fail. One wonders whether Freud perceived that, if analysis worked, this claim was redundant, and if transference worked, it might do so irrespective of any effect of analysis. Experience in other areas of human interaction has shown that it is precisely the quality of the interpersonal relationship between the participants that determines the effectiveness of any improvement in the state of the patient's mind.

Freud's 'talking cure' – psychoanalysis – remains popular with millions of people who are more interested in talking about themselves or in obtaining some kind of psychological support than in the strictly scientific merits of the procedure. Many of these people consider the fees they pay the therapist money well spent. There is no point in arguing with the proponents of psychoanalysis because they do not speak the same language as scientists so there is little common ground for discussion. It is, however, very important for people seeking such treatment to be aware that a significant proportion of seemingly psychological symptoms are due to conditions for which scientific medicine does have a cure. In some such cases, the cost of psychoanalysis may be greater than the patient realizes.

Recent developments

Recent years have seen a growing realization that there is an important link between the immune system and those brain processes concerned with thought, perception, behaviour and organic disease. We are now beginning to understand that the immune system does not work in isolation in its defence against infection, tumours and foreign material. A reflection of this awareness has been the development of a new branch of medical science known as psychoneuroimmunology. This branch is concerned with the study of the interactions between the mind and the immune system.

The link between the higher brain functions and the hormonal systems of the body has long been understood. We are now gaining a clearer understanding of the ways in which hormones can affect the immune system. These interactions begin to explain much that was previously obscure about the way that the body can respond to psychological stress. Psychoneuro-immunological research also promises advances in our understanding of how human behaviour can alter immune system function and how psychosocial factors and emotional states can affect the development of diseases such as infections and cancers.

These developments indicate that there is a closer link between psychology and disease than we have previously appreciated. While we should never underestimate the importance of human factors in medical treatment, there is much to be said for the view that what we need to combat psychological problems is more science and less pseudo-scientific dogma of the psychoanalytic variety.

The manufacture of madness

The Manufacture of Madness is the title of a remarkable book by the American psychiatrist Thomas S. Szasz (1920–). Szasz was born in Budapest but trained as a doctor in America where he also underwent postgraduate studies at the Chicago Institute for Psychoanalysis. In 1956 he was appointed Professor of Psychiatry at the State University of New York at Syracuse. He is a scholarly man who has written many books and who has published hundreds of articles and reviews, both for a professional and a lay readership.

To understand Szasz's central proposition, one must first have a general idea of the condition about which he is, naturally, most concerned – schizophrenia.

Schizophrenia is the commonest major psychiatric disorder and affects about 1 per cent of the population of the Western World. It usually shows itself before the age of twenty-five and lasts for life. About half the patients in mental hospitals are schizophrenics, as are many of the homeless who inhabit city streets. Schizophrenia is not, however, a disease in the normal medical sense and has no fixed characteristics. Definitions vary widely and the condition is constantly being officially redefined. At one time it was called 'premature dementia' (*dementia praecox*), but it is in no sense a dementia and the intellectual powers are not affected. There is no laboratory test for schizophrenia and no observable change in the nervous system. The diagnosis is based entirely on the behaviour of the person under consideration. This is an important point.

It is not easy to discuss schizophrenia in the same terms as an organic disorder as it is impossible to be as certain of the reality of 'symptoms' as with organic disease, and much must be inferred from the affected person's behaviour and statements. Schizophrenics are said to suffer from false beliefs (delusions), false sensations (hallucinations), disordered thinking, and loss of awareness of reality. They have a tendency to ramble in speech, with non-logical free associations, loss of the distinction between literal and metaphorical meaning, the use of invented words (neologisms), and unusual applications of common words.

Several theories have been proposed to account for schizophrenia. Freud taught that the disorder arose from lack of early maternal affection. Others held that it was caused by unresolved sexual or emotional conflicts. Current thinking favours the idea of social environmental stress or life experience (programming) of a kind rendering the individual incapable of relating 'normally' to society or the world in general. The finding of biochemical changes in the nervous system of schizophrenic people – excess of the neurotransmitter dopamine, for instance – by no means necessarily indicates that this is the cause of the disease. Alteration in neurotransmitter may be no more than a correlate of 'abnormal' behaviour as may be the lack of increased blood flow in the frontal lobes of the brain, shown by positron emission tomography (PET scanning), in schizophrenics.

On the other hand, since brain abnormalities can certainly cause most, if not all, of the manifestations of schizophrenia and, since brain abnormalities can result from unsatisfactory programming, or information input, during the developmental period of the nervous system, the causation may involve both external and internal factors.

The evidence of genetic studies suggests that genes exist which confer a susceptibility to the disorder. The closer the genetic relationship to a person with schizophrenia, the more likely one is to suffer the disorder oneself. Identical twins show the highest concordance rate. It should, of course, be remembered that the closer the genetic relationship, the more similar the environmental influences. There have been a few studies of identical twins one of which was reared separately from the parents. These suggest that the adopted twin is as likely to develop schizophrenia as the twin remaining with the natural parents, thereby supporting a genetic element in the causation.

Schizophrenia certainly runs in families. In the children of one schizophrenic parent the incidence is about ten per cent.

When both parents are affected, the incidence is about 50 per cent. About ten per cent of the brothers or sisters of a schizophrenic develop the condition. In the case of identical twins, the figure is about 50 per cent. But heredity cannot explain the causes of schizophrenia.

Classically, three varieties of schizophrenia are described:
• paranoid schizophrenia, with delusions usually of persecution or grandeur
• hebephrenic schizophrenia, with extreme mental disorganization, silliness of emotion and behaviour, and ideas of bodily deterioration
• catatonic schizophrenia

Catatonic schizophrenia characterised the conventional notion of 'madness'. It occurred after a long period of gradual loss of interest in life with growing apathy and indifference which drifted into stupor and a tendency to remain unmoving in one position in a state of trance-like immobility and unresponsiveness. There was parrot-like repetition of words spoken (echolalia) or imitation of actions performed (echopraxia). The affected person was said to remain unmoving, allegedly for hours, in any position in which he or she had been placed, even if the position was bizarre and awkward. The limbs displayed an odd, stiff flexibility, and the joints bent slowly but unresistingly, under pressure, into new positions. This wax-like flexibility was called *flexibilitas cerea*, which is the same thing in Latin. Food was refused and faeces retained indefinitely. There was often urinary incontinence. Every command was resisted. Such people were, however, fully aware of everything said to them and could recall the details later when, weeks or months later, there was sudden recovery.

Today, catatonic schizophrenia is very rare, and recent studies have shown that depression is a far commoner cause of catatonia than schizophrenia. That organic brain disease can cause catatonia has been viewed by some as evidence that schizophrenia is a neurological disease. Others have found that the nature of catatonia strongly suggests that, on the contrary, it is a reactive response to intolerable circumstances.

So the three-part classification described above is no longer relevant and the condition cannot be so neatly divided. Paranoid schizophrenia is still very common, hebephrenic, much less so.

Schizophrenia is treated mainly with antipsychotic drugs which, although not bringing about a cure, can, while they are being taken, usually restore the affected person to a state generally acceptable to society. Electroconvulsive therapy was widely used until the late 1950s, but was displaced by the development of the drug largactil and is now rarely employed. Largactil was the forerunner of a wide range of antipsychotic drugs. Psychoanalysis has no value in the treatment of schizophrenia.

This brief description brings out some of the major points on which Szasz bases his thesis – a thesis impressively and convincingly argued in his books *The Myth of Mental Illness* and *The Manufacture of Madness*. Essentially, Szasz argues that schizophrenia is not, in fact, a disease. The paradigm of organic disorder has been thoughtlessly, or perhaps deliberately, extended to an entity of quite a different kind. This is done so as to provide the doctors – and officialdom generally – with the power to deal oppressively with people who do not conform to the majority view of how people should behave. Szasz points out that this is not a new phenomenon. Exactly the same kind of punitive attitude was taken, until about 300 years ago, to people who were also deemed to be breaking the rules. Then, society created, and punished, witches; today society creates, and punishes, schizophrenics. In both cases, the punishment included stigmatization, denial of legal rights, loss of liberty, incarceration and enforced treatment. In both cases the response has involved legalized murder. In both cases, what is done is done for that person's 'own good'.

If a person finds his or her situation so intolerable that an alternative world is desperately needed, are we entitled to deny them that refuge? The retreat into a world of one's own making – a comfortable place in which none of the horrors of 'real life' exist – may be the only alternative to suicide that many unfortunates have. Are we entitled to force them to take drugs or other forms of treatment that, in effect, drag them back into our world?

Szasz argues his case very convincingly. Whatever arguments one may adduce to counter his position – and there are many strong points to be made – these arguments are not scientific. Szasz's view is strongly at variance with that of the medical Establishment. Both cannot be right.

Clearly there is a blunder somewhere.

Chapter 7

Human guinea pigs

Human guinea pigs in Nazi Germany

Doctors have almost always wanted to experiment with their ideas on humans themselves. On the few occasions when they have been allowed to do so the results have generally been catastrophic.

'In one instance,' said the witness Walter Neff, who as an inmate of Dachau had assisted Dr Rascher throughout his research, 'it was found that the heart was still beating after the chest and skull had been laid open ... this particular experiment was actually the cause of many more deaths, since tests were afterwards repeatedly made with the intention of ascertaining how long the heart of a dissected body would go on beating.'

Himmler was particularly interested in this, It raised the fascinating possibility that the dead could be recalled to life. It was actually more interesting than the data Rascher's work on high altitude and low pressure was yielding. He urged him to proceed.

Dr Sigmund Rascher, Staff Surgeon of the Luftwaffe and SS *Untersturmführer*, was an ambitious young man. The technological challenges of war, the extremities of heat, cold, height, and depth to which men were exposed provided a myriad of military research opportunities in which fast and favourable results were noticed and rewarded at the highest level. Rascher was aware that, win or lose, war could not last indefinitely; there might only be a limited period in which to make use of unique facilities and associated liberties, a few precious years in which to advance his career. He already had a reputation for haste and plagiarism in his work; he had attempted and failed commercially to exploit an experimental blood coagulant called Polygal 10, whose formula had been stolen from a Jewish chemist Rascher had encountered when he first worked in a concentration camp. That was at Dachau in 1939, and Rascher had tried his new find on some of the prisoners. It didn't work, and his guinea pigs were later shot.

Driving with his uncle three years later, on a fine summer evening near Munich, the older man, who felt a need to satisfy his conscience, invited Rascher, sitting preoccupied, and looking rather ill at ease in his snug SS uniform, to comment on the rumours surrounding his current work. To his surprise, Rascher did not deny them; in fact, he became tearful, and nearly hysterical. He said that he knew he was doing evil, but the bargain had been struck; it was too late, and there was no way back for him. He would persist with experiments on human beings.

Rascher's experiments

In 1941, Rascher, along with Luftwaffe and civilian colleagues, had been investigating the effects of high altitude and low pressure on the human body. The possibility of manufacturing jet aircraft, capable of flying at heights of over 18,000 metres (some 11 miles) made the work urgent. At their various institutions throughout Germany, doctors had tried to simulate the effects of high altitude and low pressure without oxygen on themselves, but rarely rose above 13,500 metres; it was too painful, too dangerous. 'Very severe pains in the head began,' wrote one researcher, 'as if my skull were being smashed open.' The research proceeded slowly. Rascher, who was then based in Munich, was frustrated with the minor role he was playing in these trials. He saw in the dilemma a strange opportunity; if the work were shifted to the concentration camp, where he knew great discoveries were possible, he might assume control.

His wife knew Himmler, and Rascher wrote directly to the leader of the SS. The research, he said, was being hindered by a lack of volunteers. 'Is there any possibility that two or three professional criminals might be made available for these experiments?' he inquired earnestly: 'The experiments, in which the experimental subject may of course die, would take place with my collaboration ... I had an absolutely confidential talk with the representative of the Luftwaffe physician who is conducting these experiments. He is of the opinion that the problem can only be solved by experiments on human beings (feeble-minded individuals could also be used as experimental material).'

He enclosed a photograph of his latest child.

Himmler consented, with the proviso that Rascher would be in charge. Rascher had the low-pressure chamber moved to Dachau. Soon after starting research there, with the first of the 'volunteers', a colleague called Romberg was surprised to see Rascher allowing the pressure in the chamber to drop well beyond the tolerance level of the subject, who was not equipped with oxygen for assimilated high flight. Romberg later claimed, during his trial at Nuremberg, that he demanded that Rascher stop, but that he was ignored, and then ordered not to interfere by his young superior, who, sweating and highly strung, continued to turn the tap lowering the pressure, and watched the subject pass from physical agony into a coma and the stillness of death.

'Terminal experiments'

It was Rascher who provided the world with the first known accounts of 'terminal experiments': those designed to cause the death of their subjects.

Himmler had said that convicted criminals sentenced to death should be used: Russians, Poles, and Jews. They were occasionally presented with the choice between death and experimentation, but of the two hundred or so used by Rascher, perhaps ten volunteered. At least eighty died. If they survived 'terminal' experiments and particularly if they could be recalled to life from apparent death Himmler allowed that they should be 'pardoned to concentration camp for life', a baffling notion of freedom. One subject, who endured a series of tests and refused to die, was actually released, and sent instead to an SS research unit for 'special service'.

Simulated heights of up to 21,000 metres were used in the experiments. Subjects were raised and lowered to and from this height, created through a low-pressure vacuum, both with and without oxygen. 'Terminal' experiments not only yielded information about the extent of human tolerance, they also allowed for subsequent dissection, so that the physiological effects of lack of oxygen and low pressure could be studied. It was while raising a subject to an extreme height that Rascher realized that the heart continued to beat after the apparent death of the subject.

Himmler had founded a pseudo-scientific body known as the Ancestral Heritage Committee. Dedicated to creating a specific SS medicine, this *mélange* of antiquarians, mystics, scientists, historians, and philosophers was an influential but hopelessly disorganised body, which interfered at will in the work of others. It was particularly interested in anything with occult overtones. It was to Himmler and this body that Rascher addressed his letter on the death of a subject. This, despite the mixture of latent enthusiasm, and neutral scientific observation, describes the death of a human being. Rascher's testament to his own feelings obscures our view of those whose emotions went unchronicled; horribly, the only way we have of knowing victims is in perceiving the world through Rascher's eyes: 'The third experiment was so extraordinary that I called an SS physician of the camp as a witness ... It was a continuous experiment without oxygen at a height of 12 km, conducted on a thirty-seven-year-old Jew in good condition. Breathing continued up to thirty minutes. After four minutes he began to perspire and to wiggle his head, after five minutes cramps occurred, between six and ten minutes breathing increased in pace and he became unconscious, from eleven to thirty minutes breathing slowed down to three breaths per minute and finally stopped altogether... severe cyanosis developed in between and foam appeared at the mouth ... about half an hour after breathing had stopped, dissection was started.'

The experiments, initially justified on the ground of military expediency, that they might save the lives of German airmen, were now driven by sheer curiosity, by a morbid interest in locating the precise point of death, by a desire to open up a few corpses while one had the opportunity. Rascher was pleasing his master.

Later, at the Nuremberg trials in 1946, various complex philosophical and moral justifications of their conduct were advanced by the twenty German doctors charged. Not one of them offered half an apology. Typical was Dr Gerhardt Rose, who had experimented with typhus on inmates and whose main concern was for his professional reputation. 'I hope, therefore,' he declared, sloshing around in self-pity, 'that my desire for my honour at least to be left to me will be recognized as natural.'

Some of what was said at Nuremberg will emerge in more detail as this chapter progresses, so far-reaching have its implications been. But the main thrust of the defence was that there were historic precedents for experimentation on human beings; that under the circumstances of war, the Germans had no choice; and that it was only undertaken in the belief that they were serving a greater good. They stressed the compulsion, moral and physical, under which they laboured, and it is worth quoting from the defence offered by Doctor Fritz Fischer, Waffen SS *Sturmbannführer*, sentenced to life imprisonment: 'We could no longer see ourselves as independent of our national destiny. The external propaganda implied that we were like the crew of a ship in a storm ... every individual fate was bound up with that of all. I am sure it was this argument that persuaded many to adopt loyal, unquestioning obedience to the Führer, no longer as a Party Leader ... but as head of the German Reich. Thus the whole position in 1942 had become that of a life or death struggle ... we did not regard ourselves as anything but German citizens of a state depending for its organization on unqualified and absolute obedience to orders given from above. We could only do our duty as responsible people by our compliance with instructions ... how spiritually and morally binding that law of war became, simply because we found that in obedience to a fulfilment of it, our friends and soldiers, both known and unknown to us, laid down their lives. I discovered in attempting to account philosophically for this situation that it cannot be understood by the individual, because it is beyond the grasp of one mind, on the level, that is, of the State ... the individual must comply with the orders of the State ... it was forced upon us. Such is the tragedy to which my generation was exposed. It would not be right to complain of it, because then I should be complaining of having been born a German.' He went on to argue that in a philosophical sense, the State was the instrument of the 'Divine Will', and in obeying it they had simply been obeying the God they knew, who through the destiny of the State wove history.

The Nazi doctor, dramatized as a tragic hero caught between his duty as a physician and his loyalty to his nation, driven hopelessly upon the wind of wicked propaganda, looking to the heavens for moral instruction as to what he should do, hears to his relief the voice of the State; and, no longer wrestling with his conscience, he plunges his knife into the spread-eagled, and still-conscious victim, whispering to himself, 'Now I know it is for some greater good.' His victim has played no role in his dilemma; like an actor working on a part, the doctor has been solely concerned with finding a motive for his own exceptional behaviour, and by elevating his shoddy predicament to a cosmic level, he has escaped his human responsibilities.

The ambiguous notion of a 'greater good' has provided the justification for countless reprehensible acts in the area of experimentation on humans; but leaving that, and the question of obedience to authority, aside for a moment, it is apparent that there are other explanations for the alacrity with which the

Nazi doctors turned to human experimentation.

Rascher, for example, was lying when he told Himmler that there were no German volunteers for the high altitude/low pressure experiments. There had been volunteers. But Rascher wanted to conduct terminal experiments on humans; it was the fast track to personal success. Moreover, it showed a certain eagerness, that one had shaken off the constraints of a decadent morality. And it demonstrated emotional strength, that one had the will. There was, frankly, a certain cachet attached to the process. The right to experiment on humans was not permitted to everybody; some scientists were still restricted to the primitive level of experimentation on animals.

Again, in the case of Professor and Doctor of Medicine Karl Gebhardt, Himmler's personal physician and Head of the German Red Cross, who was hanged after Nuremberg, personal ambition and professional rivalry were the principal motivations. When Heydrich, the personal favourite of Hitler, was assassinated in Prague in May 1942, Gebhardt had advocated certain surgical measures to save his life. These had been neglected in favour of techniques proposed by Morrell, Hitler's personal physician. Gebhardt was stung by the rejection, and after Heydrich's death sought to prove that had he been listened to, Heydrich would have survived. To demonstrate the efficacy of his methods, he wrested control of research into bone transplantation and the use of sulphonamide anti-bacterial drugs that was at the time being conducted at Ravensbrück with the ostensible object of finding ways of treating the terrible injuries occurring on the Russian front. Here, along with the philosophically minded Dr Fischer, Gebhardt created artificial wounds in the bodies of drugged and blindfolded female prisoners, for authenticity inserting shards of glass, earth, wood and metal splinters, applied ligatures to limbs and infected the wounds with tetanus, so that the drugs (applied externally) could be tested. The women became mere carriers, breeding grounds for the bacteria Gebhardt wished to study, and when he examined them, he looked only with pride and frustration at the little colonies he had founded on their legs. Then he began to dabble in bone transplantation, smashing limbs with a hammer to see how they might be repaired by bone grafting, and taking the shoulder blade of an insane man and inserting it into a healthy prisoner. He conducted experiments on nerve and muscle regeneration. Afterwards, the men and women he had so tortured were killed by fatal injections of benzine.

In passing judgement on him, the Nuremberg Tribunal stated that he 'had not been ordered to carry out the experiments, but on the contrary had sought the opportunity to do so'. In this, he was not alone.

Dr Sigmund Rascher did not survive to be tried at Nuremberg. His ambitions turned to dust, and he was consumed by the monsters he so passionately tried to appease with human sacrifices. Himmler had him hanged at Dachau in 1944; his wife died in another concentration camp.

One of the formal charges against the Nazi doctors was that they acted without the consent of their subjects. Since a pragmatic strand of the Nazi defence had been that there were precedents for human experimentation without consent, and precedents for those experiments involving condemned 'criminals' who had been offered remission of their sentences as a reward for participating in tests, the Nuremberg Tribunal felt it necessary, in concluding its judgements, to offer to the world the first formal guidelines intended to preserve the legal rights of the patient. It was deeply ironic that it should have been actions by Germans that prompted this, as in 1931 Germany had passed strict laws against medical and scientific abuse of individuals, laws which the Nazis had never bothered to repeal.

It is these ethical guidelines stated at Nuremberg that form the basis of our modern theory of 'informed consent'. It is the 'informed consent' of the individual to a treatment that preserves his or her status, and rights as a patient.

The tribunal held that the 'voluntary consent of the human subject is absolutely essential,' and this required that the person involved should have a legal capacity to give consent (that they should not be mentally incapacitated, or be a minor, for example), that they must be in a position to have freedom of choice, without duress (no prisoners under sentence of death), and that they should have 'sufficient knowledge and comprehension of the elements of the subject to make an understanding and enlightened decision' (they must not be manipulated by complex medical language or blinded with science).

Other points in the statement attempted to define under what circumstances experimentation on humans was permissible, and under what conditions the work should be conducted. There was one overriding stipulation: that the scientist in charge must be prepared to abandon the experiment if it 'is likely to result in injury, disability or death to the experimental subject.'

The principle of the 'greater good', advanced to justify the medical murder of the individual was considered irrelevant.

Out of the darkness of Nuremberg came this point of light, which was then enshrined in the Helsinki Declaration of 1961. Here a distinction was made between 'therapeutic' and 'non-therapeutic' research on humans. The latter was outlawed.

Every time a doctor treats a patient it is an experiment; to be engaged in a 'therapeutic' encounter, the doctor must hold the health of his patient as his primary objective. 'Therapeutic' research, therefore, was defined as 'research combined with patient care' and justified by its 'potential' healing value to the patient. Informed consent was required, but a loophole was left; consent might not be necessary if it was 'not consistent with patient psychology', in other words, if knowing the truth might, in the view of the doctor, damage the patient's chances.

Human experimentation in postwar America

The guidelines established at Nuremberg and Helsinki gradually became the ethical basis of most branches of medicine and science, or should have done. However, within a few years of the Second World War, there was an unprecedented upsurge in largely unprincipled human experimentation. The discredited, arrogant and hopelessly general notion of the 'greater good' appeared again. The massive expansion of the pharmaceutical industry, which flooded the market with new products in the 1950s, and the new fashion for chemical treatment, ensured that greater good and greater profits became interchangeable ideas. Surgical techniques had been given a huge boost by the expediency of war, but the end of hostilities brought restrictions on research; doctors and scientists looked for areas where 'informed consent' could be manipulated.

Experiments on prisoners
Prisoners provided the largest captive testing group. By 1960, it was estimated that 20,000 federal prisoners in the USA were

Sigmund Rascher also performed experiments with prolonged supercooling on prisoners at Dachau. Due to the great number of airmen lost over the North Sea it was considered urgent to find ways of reviving those who had been exposed to freezing temperatures. Rascher favoured an orthodox approach to his research: immersing drugged prisoners (conscious ones shouted too loudly, which upset him) in freezing water, or leaving them outside, naked, in the snow, and then seeing how quickly, if at all, they could be revived through immersion in hot water (the heart stops quickly at low temperatures). But Himmler, with his usual interest in the arcane, expressed an interest in seeing whether there were any native German folk-remedies, such as herbal teas used by good Aryan fishermen, which might have mysterious powers. Moreover, he was convinced that animal warmth would revive frozen and near-dead men more quickly than hot water; he could imagine a fisherman's wife 'taking her frozen husband to bed'. If Himmler insisted, Rascher would oblige, and quickly. Hence several women prisoners were procured and forced, naked, into bed with the frozen victims with orders to revive them. These experiments provided nothing other than tragic and absurd sex scenes for the watching Germans. In regretfully telling Himmler that hot water was still the most efficient means of revival, Rascher added that he would like to move operations to Auschwitz, where the climate was colder, and where, in a bigger camp, less attention would be drawn to his work. 'For the subjects howl so when they freeze!' he wrote.

Other experiments conducted throughout the concentration camps, in which doctors participated, included tests on the possibility of drinking sea-water, and trials of phosgene and mustard gas, in which subjects were made to inhale the substances, after they had been given ampoules of gas and ordered to smash them, and endure them being applied directly to their skin in five-day or six-day experiments which resulted in appalling burns, blindness and inevitable if prolonged death. The bodies from the gas tests were then sent to the Ancestral Heritage Committee for dissection. Here witnesses described the manner in which the internal organs – the lungs and intestines of the victims – had been almost entirely rotted away.

Inmates were also used in quite dreadful experiments to determine the fastest means to sterilize whole populations of 'undesirables' without diminishing their capacity for slave labour. It was also hoped that, ideally, a manner would be found in which the victim would not be aware as to what was happening. Naturally, this was an area in which Hitler took a great personal interest and there was no shortage of eager proposals from doctors, all advocating their own methods. Later they would claim as did Viktor Brack, who was hanged, that they were actually trying to save the lives of these people. If they were sterilized, they would be saved from execution. The methods tried included castration of the males, which was found to be too time-consuming, the injection of caustic solutions into the ovaries of women, again too fiddly a process, and the use of radiation on the genitals of male prisoners. This was to be surreptitiously administered by a concealed device while the prisoners were standing at a desk filling in forms. At the experimental stage, subjects were simply irradiated, and their testicles then amputated for examination of the effects; the subjects were then killed, if they had not died already. This was part of the overall ideology of 'eugenics', which besides the genocide in the camps included the state 'euthanasia' plan to eliminate the occupants of German mental hospitals through gassing them in roving vans. Research into typhus, hepatitis and malaria was conducted at Buchenwald, Natzweiler and Sachsenhausen camps by a number of honourable doctors, all vying for the opportunity of being the first to discover vaccines. The typhus experiments were driven along by Himmler, who wanted a 'Special SS' vaccine for his beloved butchers fighting on the eastern front. At Buchenwald, in one period in 1942, some nineteen kinds of vaccine were tried out on 481 prisoners, a quarter of whom died during or shortly after the experiments. Many of the doctors involved in these abominations were hanged, shot or imprisoned before Nuremberg or as a consequence of other trials; Mitscherlich and Mielke, the two German doctors who first chronicled the revelations of Nuremberg for a disbelieving world in their book *The Death Doctors*, estimated that there were 350 German doctors engaged in such activities.

* * * * *

Experiments on soldiers

While the Nazis flagrantly used innocent prisoners for mass experimentation, other nations have experimented on their own troops. The effects of radiation and anthrax were observed on British soldiers. American veterans of Vietnam have been claiming for years that they were used in trials of 'psychotropic' (mind-altering) drugs, and thousands of other veterans were affected by experimental chemical defoliants. The most recent use of troops in experimentation to come to light is the forced participation of American sailors in mustard gas tests in 1943. Then, within sight of the dome of the White House in Washington, seventeen-year-old naval novices, many of whom had been told that they were going to test a new range of summer uniforms for the navy, were thrust into a gas chamber and engulfed with mustard and arsenic-based gases. It was not until March 1993, after fifty years of silence, that the US Navy finally released details of its 'man-break' experiments, in which 2,500 US sailors were used in gas tests. Driven by fears that the Germans and Japanese were about to use poison gas, the Americans needed to develop and test better clothing and masks. The US Army would not allow its troops to be used (they remembered all too well the effects of mustard gas in the First World War, when it caused 400,000 casualties). The Navy, on the other hand, volunteered its men, who were compelled to undergo the tests by threats of court martial and forty years' imprisonment. The Navy's official documents of the period noted that 'occasionally there have been individuals or groups who have refused to co-operate fully. A short explanatory talk and if necessary a slight verbal dressing down have always proved satisfactory.'

The research, which crippled the lungs and shortened the lives of hundreds, was pointless. No gas was used in the war except by the Allies, and then by accident, when a boatload that Churchill ordered to Italy was bombed off Bari. The gas escaped and killed over a thousand local civilians. In keeping with the customs of war, Churchill had the whole unpleasant matter expunged from the record. No mention was made of mustard gas, and the deaths were put down to enemy action. As for the American sailors who joined up to fight for their country only to be told that they could be of more use being gassed by their country, they have faced a fifty-year battle for compensation for the injuries inflicted on them.

participating as 'volunteers' in medical experiments. Prisoners, because of their regimented lifestyle and restricted movements, made excellent testing fodder. They were easy to persuade and easy to monitor. In 1963, it was found that the medical director of the Oklahoma State Penitentiary had made a series of deals with drug companies permitting them to test their products on prisoners. For volunteering, the prisoners received a small payment, while the doctors involved were grossing up to $300,000 a year. At Ohio State Prison, inmates were injected with live cancer cells and in Chicago they had the blood of leukaemia sufferers pumped into them. Neither group would contract the diseases, but that was not known when the research was undertaken; the object was to see whether such fatal sicknesses could be transmitted.

At Holmsburg Prison in Pennsylvania, nine out of ten prisoners were volunteering for medical experimentation in return for a small payment. The prison even had special cells which were made available to the researchers. Here, new chemical products, new techniques and experimental drugs were tried out. *Time* magazine revealed that the federal government was sponsoring medical research in fifteen out of thirty-seven penal institutions. Federal prisoners were offered rewards ranging from a packet of cigarettes to $25 in cash; and if the experiment was, in the estimation of the prison authorities, a serious one involving risk to the subject, the prisoner might receive 'meritorious good-time credits'; a few days scrapped off the sentence.

One American scientist was heard to say: 'Criminals in our penitentiaries are fine experimental material and much cheaper than chimpanzees.'

The Nuremberg guidelines had specifically warned against testing in such captive populations. The Nazi doctors had naturally argued that their victims had been branded 'criminals' by the almighty State, and the Nuremberg Tribunal had noted that such 'labelling' was a significant part of the insidious process of dehumanising individuals, by which they were transformed into laboratory specimens. The Americans had been among the first to apply as a legal principle the lesson of Nuremberg that consent should be obtained. But prisoners remained particularly vulnerable to promises of remission which quite overwhelmed rational judgement in much the same way that a threat would. Other subtle encouragements to participate were also made, ranging from the loss of privileges through simple bribery to moral blackmail (this was an opportunity to serve society). In contrast, the morality of their testers was never scrutinised before they were let loose on the prisoners.

Nor were the mentally sick and defective spared in peace time. Once again, it was claimed their consent had been obtained. But in all the cases it was debatable as to whether they had been capable of providing consent, and whether they had understood the implications of the experiments – if, indeed, any attempt had been made to explain them. Whereas prisons provided adults, the attraction with testing on the mentally defective was the availability of large groups of children in institutions.

In 1962, in America, fifty 'juvenile delinquents' and mentally handicapped teenagers were used to test a new antibiotic which was supposed to target acne. Within a fortnight half of them had liver damage, though this did not stop the researchers who were pleased to note that, as expected, jaundice followed. The children were also subjected to liver puncture needles on a number of occasions (a horrendously dangerous and painful process). When they got better, they were made ill again to check the effects of the drug. Around the same time, researchers in England used fifty-six mentally handicapped children in trials of a measles vaccine. Many subsequently suffered from complex rashes and one developed broncho-pneumonia.

In America, twelve infants aged from one to nine months old who were mentally handicapped by hydrocephalus were used in research into cerebro-spinal fluid which was in no way related to their illness. Following injection with a radioactive compound, needles were inserted through the skull, through the back of the neck and into the lumbar spine to tap off cerebro-spinal fluid. Mentally defective infants with no history of abnormality in their calcium metabolism were administered with radioactive compounds in studies on calcium metabolism; and radioactive iodine compounds were given to another nineteen mentally handicapped children in tests on iodine metabolism.

The above instances are only a sample of the practices that were common in the post-war years. Two important books did much to expose what the medical establishment were doing – Beacher's *Experimentation on Man,* and Pappworth's *Human Guinea Pigs* – but many people refused to believe that this conduct could be so widespread while the world was still in the shadow of the Nazi death camps. Yet, most extraordinarily, most of the experiments which Beacher and Pappworth recounted had been detailed in the medical press, as is the accepted process for any new work seeking recognition. The public, however, do not read the medical press, and even for those who do, it can be hard to imagine, in the description of an experiment, what precisely is happening to the human subject; the language of science does not reflect pain, bewilderment and anger. It records only a series of interesting phenomena that flicker across its gaze; its only emotion is enthusiasm for its own process.

There was a lack of public reportage of deaths and mishaps in experimentation and even in everyday treatment. Unfavourable details were habitually omitted from reports. In two frequent procedures, the liver biopsy performed by needle and trans-lumbar aortography, it was admitted that deaths were far more frequent than had been recorded. In the latter operation, the patient was turned on to his or her face and a large needle stabbed into the back at one side of the spinal column, penetrating to a depth of six inches so that it pierced the wall of the abdominal aorta, the main artery to the abdominal organs and the lower limbs. As the needle entered the aorta, blood spurted back into the needle. A contrast medium was then injected so that the aorta and its branches could be observed by X-ray. In 1957 a leading American radiologist, who knew of the dangers of the operation and was puzzled by the infrequency of reported deaths, wrote to 450 radiologists. He received replies from only 194 of them. These replies revealed thirty-seven deaths directly attributable to this common but recently introduced procedure, and another ninety-eight cases of serious non-fatal injury, including twenty-four cases where paralysis of both legs had ensued. All this – and this could not have been the whole story – had gone unremarked in the medical press.

The confusion over medical ethics and the question of 'informed consent' in experimentation spilled over into other areas of the human sciences. In particular psychology, often reliant on the ignorance of its human subjects, came under scrutiny following Milgram's famous tests on human obedience.

This story takes us back to the Nazis. For Milgram, who was accused of practicing in a manner deemed ethically reprehensible, was actually inspired to carry out his investigations into human obedience after he had read transcripts of the Nuremberg trials and literature on the Holocaust. In these accounts, he noted that individuals who considered themselves human were capable of performing the most unspeakable acts if commanded to do so by those in authority, whether because they were genuinely frightened, simply trained in obedience or felt that the responsibility for their actions lay not with them, but with those who gave the orders. Milgram wanted to test obedience to and defiance of authority in ordinary citizens. In his tests, active deception of the subjects was essential.

He advertised in newspapers inviting subjects to participate in 'a study of memory and learning'. He recruited subjects with varied levels of education, of varied social standing and from different occupations, between the ages of 20 and 50. There were paid $4 (plus 50c travel expenses) for an hour of participation in the 'study'.

At the first stage, Milgram took two people into a psychology laboratory to participate in what he said bluntly was a 'memory experiment'. One of these two would be a naïve subject, someone who had replied to his advertisement. The other was an accomplice, who passed himself off as another naïve subject. In the laboratory the researcher explained the study to them. One of the two – the genuine subject – was to be deemed the 'teacher'; Milgram's disguised accomplice would be the 'learner'. The subject was now told that the experiment was specifically concerned with the effects of punishment upon the learning process.

In an adjacent room, out of sight, he was told, there was an 'electric chair' apparatus. To this the 'learner' was apparently led and strapped. The 'teacher' was told that the researcher would conduct a series of word association tests on the hidden 'learner'. Every time he got an answer wrong, he would be punished by an electric shock. It would be the 'teacher's' job to administer that shock as and when requested by the researcher. The 'teacher' was then seated at an imposing electrical shock generator. Its range went from 15 to 450 volts. In front of the 'teacher' were a series of labelled voltage settings. These ascended from 'slight shock' through to 'moderate shock', 'strong shock', 'very strong shock', 'intense shock', 'extreme intense shock', 'danger; severe shock' and, finally, an ambiguous 'xxx'. To acquaint them with the feeling of a slight shock, the 'teacher' was exposed to a fifteen-volt shock before the start of the experiment proper.

Then the researcher began to ask the 'learner' questions. Each time he got one wrong, the 'teacher' was required to administer shocks of increasing intensity. Of course, the man in the other room was not being hurt, but the guinea pig could not know this. The 'learner' completed the deception by sound: at 75 volts he grunted; at 120 volts he shouted and complained; from 150 volts he demanded to be released; at 270 volts he began screaming; at 300 volts he fell silent.

'Teachers' reacted in various ways, of course, but typically, when the 'learner' first started complaining they would ask the researcher if they should continue. At this, and every subsequent expression of doubt, the researcher would aggressively state that it was absolutely essential that the experiment continue, and that although the shocks were painful they were not dangerous. The study was necessary for the advancement of science.

The 'teacher' would begin to show distinct signs of conflict between a reluctance to inflict pain and an instinct to obey authority. As the voltage and audible evidence of pain increased, so did their anguish. Milgram noted how rapidly a human could disintegrate under these circumstances. 'I observed,' he wrote, 'a mature and poised businessman enter the laboratory smiling and confident. Within twenty minutes he was reduced to a stuttering wreck who was rapidly approaching the point of nervous collapse.'

The experiment was concluded when either the maximum voltage was reached or the 'teacher' adamantly refused to go any further.

Astonishingly, Milgram found that, despite their apparent reluctance, approximately 60 per cent of subjects were fully obedient to the authority of the researcher and punished the 'learner' right up to the 'xxx' on the voltage indicator.

Afterwards, the subjects had the deception explained to them and met the 'learner'. They were questioned as to why they had continued to administer shocks. The typical response was that they could not have done it by themselves; but here, they were simply doing what they were told.

Milgram's research was published in 1963, and met with acclaim and controversy. For some, it threw light on previously incredible statements made at the Nuremberg trials. Others said the results were highly speculative and only possible within the laboratory. They posed more questions than answers. What satisfaction do we derive from seeing these statistics? Does our desire to find an explanation for the behaviour of the Nazis override our compassion for the victims? What precisely do Milgram's figures demonstrate? That 60 per cent of us are potential Nazis? How is this information useful rather than simply being impressive? Many of these questions could apply to the results of much other research on humans.

Because Milgram had not obtained – indeed, could not obtain – informed consent, he was accused of the very cruelty he was attempting to evaluate. The case led to the American Psychological Association acknowledging that deception – lying to the subject despite its possible disturbing consequences – had become virtually standard procedure in American psychology, which had grown so strongly that it was transforming that nation into a huge psychological testing laboratory. Deception was being used in at least 30 per cent of all tests. Lying was being enshrined as a prerogative, which seemed a curious state of affairs for a profession claiming to pursue the truth.

Experimentation on humans finally bubbled to the surface of American life in the early 1970s. One of the biggest scandals to emerge was that of the Tuskagee Syphilis Study, a notorious example of the sustained violation of patients' rights, carried out with the full sanction of the authorities.

The origins of the project remain murky, but it appears to have been a public health study commenced in 1932 with the stated purpose of comparing the health and longevity of an untreated and syphilitic population with a non-syphilitic but otherwise similar group. The site chosen for the study was Tuskagee in Mississippi, and the syphilitic subjects were originally 400 black males. Conceived as a short-term project, to last 6–8 months, it evolved into one of the longest studies in history, and an early fall-off in funding quickly shifted the emphasis from treating the subjects to merely observing them.

For the next thirty years, doctors simply watched people die. The syphilis sufferers, all poor and with a low standard of education, were told neither the name nor the nature of their disease, and had no idea they were 'participating' in a prolonged experiment to which they had not given their consent. It would, of course, have been impossible to conduct such research among a white population. The subjects were manipulated into attending the clinic to be examined and have regular blood samples taken by being told they were receiving free treatment for 'bad blood', a term local blacks associated with a host of unrelated ailments. They were not receiving any treatment whatsoever. The researchers assumed that by exploiting the deprivation of the population and their deference to authority and respect for medical expertise, they could persuade them to obey without questions; they even submitted subjects to regular spinal taps, which were described as a 'special free treatment'.

By 1936, it was evident that the infected subjects had twice as many health problems as the healthy subjects, and by 1946 it was clear that syphilis sufferers had a death rate twice that of the others. What more could be learned? Still the project was persisted with; still the surviving sufferers were kept in ignorance and left untreated. Such treatment as they did receive came from doctors not connected with the study who were shocked to hear of what was happening. Where possible, the researchers actually prevented the subjects from receiving effective treatment, threatening to stop their 'free medicine' for the 'bad blood', and met protest from sickening subjects with blunt lies that proper treatment was being administered; in fact, they said, their 'wonder drugs' were a 'never to be repeated opportunity'. The research had its funding reviewed, successfully, several times, and no fewer than thirteen official articles on it were published in the scientific press between 1936 and

1970. In 1972, the *New York Times* published a front page exposé of the research, and thereafter the justifications for continuing it melted away.

The lessons of these dramatic incidents of human experimentation are finally tested on us all in the disarmingly simple atmosphere of the doctor's consulting room. In March 1993 a white doctor in Zimbabwe was found to have conducted some 550 'pain control experiments' on 500 patients over a six-year period. He was particularly interested in the effects of morphine overdoses on black women, and three patients died. The case has a familiar ring to it. An extreme instance of the neglect of 'informed consent', perhaps, but a valid example of the potential for abuse in the trusting confines of an everyday doctor-patient relationship. It is only the right to consent that distinguishes the patient from the guinea pig.

Eugenics in America

Mrs E.H. Harriman

In February 1910, Charles Davenport, professional American scientist, graduate in natural history and champion of the science of good breeding – eugenics – had lunch with a wealthy lady, Mrs E. H. Harriman, widow of a railroad magnate. They had been introduced by her daughter, Mary, who had liberal beliefs and mistakenly thought that Davenport's eugenics might be a means of improving the lot of the common man. The lunch was a success for Davenport: a 'Red Letter Day for Humanity', he wrote in his diary. In retrospect, it was actually rather a bad lunch for mankind.

Mrs Harriman was to contribute half a million dollars to

finance Davenport's dream: the amassing of mountains of data on the hereditary characteristics of the American nation, to chart ' the great strains of human protoplasm coursing through the country'. Over the next few years Davenport's teams of workers scoured the country, conducting door to door interviews, sending out and analysing questionnaires, scrutinizing the public and private records of the inhabitants of prisons, poorhouses, asylums, hospitals and institutions for the mentally deficient, deaf and blind – not to see how the lives of society's marginalised, poor and sick could be improved, but to find out to what extent they had polluted the blood of the nation. Above all, the apostle-workers spread the gospel of eugenics.

By 1914, some thirty American states had marriage laws which either declared the marriages of idiots or the insane invalid, or restricted or forbade marriage among the unfit and 'feeble-minded'. Some states were ahead of others; Indiana had since 1905 forbidden the marriage of the mentally deficient, persons with 'a transmissible disease' and alcoholics. By 1917, sterilization and in some cases castration of the insane, the epileptic, the criminal, the drug-taker, the sexual offender and the catch-all 'feeble-minded' was on the statute books of sixteen states. Down in Indiana, they had been practicing such eugenic measures since 1907, even sterilizing asylum inmates for being 'persistent masturbators'. From 1907 to 1928 a little under 9,000 'unfit' members of the population were sterilized to prevent them breeding: far too few for the impatient priests of the eugenics movement, who thought there must be at least 300,000 unsuitable specimens at loose in society. In 1924 President Calvin Coolidge, who as vice-president had said that 'America must be kept American; biological laws show that Nordics deteriorate when mixed with other races',

At Nuremberg, the Nazi doctors cited precedents of experiments on condemned 'criminals', many of which had been conducted in America. Two of these were an attempt to discover a cure for pellagra, a deadly disease marked by shrivelled skin, wasting and insanity, and experiments with malaria cures. In the former case, a Professor Goldberger had in 1915 induced the disease in twelve Mississippi convicts who became seriously ill as a consequence. Before the experiment, agreements had been drawn up with the convicts' lawyers, in which they had been offered parole or release if they survived the potentially fatal experiment. In the case of the malaria research, two large sets of inmates in Chicago, and in New Jersey were used in 1944. At Stateville Prison, 441 convicts participated. A lengthy notice had been posted in the prison. It described the nature of the research and the potential risks involved, and in return for favourable consideration of their sentences and cash payments, the men were required to sign a form in which they effectively resigned all their legal rights of redress. 'I hereby accept all risks connected with the experiment,' ran the document, which proceeded to absolve everyone, from the basic researchers to the Government of the State of Illinois, from any complaint arising from the research. In the accounts of the research, it is revealed that the doses of malaria administered were close to the 'estimated maximum tolerated dose'. Many of the inmates became seriously ill, not only from the malaria, but from the effects of the experimental drugs then tried on them. They endured severe internal pains, nausea, vomiting, cyanosis (when the skin turns blue), heart trouble, drug-induced fevers, dermatitis and fluctuating blood pressure. In a third experiment cited by the Nazis, which was conducted at the beginning of the century in the Philippines, a future Professor of Tropical Medicine at Harvard University obtained permission from the Governor of the country to infect with the plague a group of men condemned to death. They knew nothing of the experiment. Later, the same professor induced beriberi, with its attendant symptoms of paralysis, mental disorder and heart trouble, in another group of prisoners, one of whom died. For this service to mankind, they were rewarded with a small gift of tobacco.

* * * * *

Experiments on cancer patients

In the mid-1950s, terminal cancer patients became portable pathological laboratories, stuck full as pincushions with catheters, needles and investigative taps draining away their fluids for examination. Using techniques which had been refined on corpses, and which they wrote rarely caused more than 'modest pain' in the barely living, doctors used mallets to drive needles into the bone marrow of cancer patients to inject radioactive contrast solutions for X-ray purposes, and inserted six-inch needles into the liver veins of patients with 'a short life expectancy', to collect blood samples and radioactive contrast solutions in ways they would surely not have considered if the patient had been healthier. In one instance hollow six-inch needles were inserted directly into the livers of seventy-three cancer patients and catheters inserted which were kept in place for nineteen days, the researchers gratefully noting that the terminal nature of the illness enabled them to ransack the patients' bodies for their morbid secrets until the very moment of death. The inert nature of the dying and the old made them excellent subjects on which to practice passing catheters through obscure arteries into remote areas never before conquered in a living human; the breast, the buttock, the spinal cord, the spleen. Three patients died during or following this fascinating inventory of their innards in 1951. 'New techniques encounter difficulties ... ' noted the researchers.

Experiments on mental patients

In the 1960s, a former winner of the Nobel Prize for Medicine, Sir John Eades, described experiments being conducted on mental patients in the USA, in which multiple holes were made in the skull of each patient through which electrodes were passed and inserted into the brain. Over the following months, these electrodes were periodically connected up to a current and the brains of the patients subjected to substantial shocks so that the effects on their behaviours could be observed. This was in the era when psychosurgery – which includes various forms of lobotomy in which the connections between the assertive frontal lobes and the rest of the brain were cut or simply mashed – still had a grasp on the imagination of American neurosurgeons. Reflecting on the fact that the patients he had witnessed had apparently given their consent to a 'treatment' which had inflicted horrendous damage on their brains, Sir John said: 'I do not believe that in the case of the brain you can explain what you are going to do, because none of us knows enough about the brain to be able to say to a subject with assurance that this is all that it will do.' Between 1945 and 1955, some 40,000 Americans were subjected to lobotomies.

* * * * *

Sterilization of 'unsuitables' in the US

Throughout the 1930s the rate at which sterilization was used on unsuitables in America rose tenfold. Virginia, ranked number two state in the nation's sterilization league, was not a good place to find yourself unemployed. Whole families of welfare-drawing mountain-dwellers were swooped on by the authorities and taken away to be sterilized. The unemployed who were afraid of being sterilized took to the hills. 'People as a whole were very much in favour of what was going on,' said one witness to a police raid. It was not enough for those like DeJarnette, a pioneer of the Virginian eugenics movement. He urged the authorities to sterilize more, faster. 'The Germans are beating us at our own game,' he said. It was 1934.

Germany had just passed a Eugenic Sterilization Law, which allowed for the immediate sterilization of people with any form of physical or mental 'abnormality'. Within three years a quarter of a million had been sterilized. In 1939, the inevitable step to mass 'euthanasia' and mass murder was taken.

The Germans flattered the American eugenicists, telling them how much they were indebted to their pioneering work. Anglo-American eugenicists on both sides of the Atlantic responded positively to the first Nazi decrees on sterilization. They showed great courage, said the American Eugenics Society.

* * * * *

Breeding cults

American cults such as the Perfectionist Oneida Community, whose founder, John Humphrey Noyes, was opposed to monogamy, found in the crusade for good breeding a convenient justification for their polygamous societies. Monogamy, Noyes argued, ran counter to the laws of good breeding, for 'while the good man will be limited by his conscience to what the law allows, the bad man, free from moral check, will distribute his seed beyond the legal limits.' Further inspired by Galton, his cult, in which all members were in theory wedded to each other with all couplings scrupulously regulated and controlled, embarked on a programme of controlled eugenic breeding.

signed the Immigration Act to limit, in the words of one Democratic Congressman, 'the alien stream ... purifying and keeping pure the blood of America'.

Within a few years the creed of eugenics, preached by men and women, doctors, scientists, mathematicians and radical social reformers, often with the best intentions, spawned the concentration camp, the gas chamber and the experiments of Dr Mengele. The grateful words that Davenport sent to Mrs Harriman after that lunch now have a horribly apposite ring. 'What a fire you have kindled!' he wrote, 'It is going to be a purifying conflagration some day!'

By the mid-1930s, it was clear to any scientist with a rational, human sensibility, that eugenics had become a perverted, black science. It was, as the American geneticist and Nobel Prize Laureate Hermann Muller said, a mere façade for 'advocates of race and class prejudice, defenders of vested interests of church and state, Fascists, Hitlerites and reactionaries generally'. It was a disaster for mankind. It had begun in a different spirit, but looking at the individuals who carried the torch, one can recognize a fatal desire for the reassuring but false certainties that eugenics offered. The certainty was in the end no more than the comfortable reinforcement of one's own prejudices.

Eugenics in England

Francis Galton, who gave us the word 'eugenics', was in many ways a typical Victorian, convinced of the importance of his age and equating the advances of the industrial revolution and the mastery of nature with the inexorable progress of man.

Galton published his ideas on good breeding in 1865, long before he had even coined the word 'eugenics'. His theories appeared in a two-part article in *Macmillan's Magazine*, which he later expanded in a book, published in 1869, entitled *Hereditary Genius*. The Victorian era abounded with biographical dictionaries of eminent men, considered exemplary reading for the young. From these Galton selected a cross-section of personages whom he considered to possess 'those qualifications of intellect and disposition which lead to reputation' in order to investigate the origins of 'natural ability'. He examined the family trees of soldiers, statesmen, poets, painters and musicians and found that an unusually large proportion of them were blood relatives. From this, Galton confidently asserted that it would be quite possible to produce a race of exceptionally gifted men by 'judicious marriages during several generations.' Galton thought such a scheme highly desirable, even necessary. The increased complexity of life in the nineteenth century required genius.

Galton proposed that there be government-sponsored competitions in hereditary merit and that the pool of winners be married off to each other in mass ceremonies at Westminster Abbey; these blessed ones would be encouraged to spawn gifted offspring by the inducement of grants. He later added the suggestion that the state should also grade the population according to their ability, permitting the higher grades to have more children than the talentless dunces at the bottom of the ladder. The inferior elements would be sequestered in monasteries and convents, and would gradually die out.

Galton erroneously equated reputation with ability. All ages have their role models, but their success is no certificate of genius. As for social advantage and disadvantage – the majority of Galton's elite were naturally the products of hereditary wealth and superior educational environments – he would have none of it. He was utterly opposed to the removal of social barriers, and preposterously used America (then not a hundred years old, its inhabitants still too busy shooting each other to pick up a pen) as an example of the corrupting effects of egalitarian thought. There 'the education of their middle and lower classes is far more advanced; but, for all that, America does certainly not exceed us in first class works of literature, art and poetry.' Educate the masses, he said, and you get quantity, not quality; America had been ninety years a nation and still produced no Shakespeare.

Francis Galton

Francis Galton, a cousin of Charles Darwin, was born in 1822, into a Midlands family. Their substantial wealth came from manufacturing guns, and Galton's father enhanced their finances with his banking skill. The Galton clan was climbing the social ladder in the prescribed fashion of the industrial revolution: first make money in manufacturing; then buy or marry a higher respectability, or win it through changing to a more suitable profession – medicine or the law.

Francis Galton was a precocious child who could read aged two and by eight was browsing through Latin texts. He knew what his father expected of him and duly went to medical school in London, but found that he hated studying medicine and suffered from perpetual headaches. He went to Cambridge and read mathematics instead, but then had a nervous breakdown, obtained a bad degree and ended up returning, unenthusiastically, to medicine.

His father died at a young age, which made Francis wealthy

and removed the need for him to pursue a respectable career. He chucked it all in and went off to Egypt, subsequently acquiring a taste for travel which left him ill at ease in conventional surroundings. Galton, whose mind was, in the words of one contemporary, 'mathematical and statistical with little or no imagination', became passionately fond of measuring things. The Victorians generally were obsessed with measuring and classifying, but Galton was exceptional. He often said: Whenever you can, count. He did not sit back and enjoy the sea and sun on his travels; he assaulted the scenery with his callipers, ruler and sextant.

From Africa he wrote to his eldest brother, noting, with considerable enjoyment, the pleasing shape of Hottentot women. 'I have seen figures that would drive the females of our land desperate – figures that could afford to scoff at crinoline.' Galton sat at a distance, using his sextant to measure their ample charms. The maps, observations and anecdotes he brought back from his expeditions made his initial reputation. After the success of *Hereditary Genius*, Galton realized that too little was known about the laws of heredity to guarantee that his envisaged super-marriages would necessarily produce supreme offspring. If eugenics was to become a reality it would need a scientific basis. He spent the rest of his life doing something then quite unique: employing the infant science of statistics to analyse the characteristics of humans in order to prove his arguments. He was ultimately awarded the highest honours by the Royal Society, and knighted in 1909.

Throughout his life, Galton suffered emotional difficulties. He was troubled by dizzy spells, headaches and various degrees of nervous breakdown, which was quite the thing among nineteenth-century intellectuals. He explained it later thus: 'Men who leave their mark on the world are very often those, who being gifted and full of nervous power, are at the same time haunted and driven by a dominant idea and are therefore within a measurable distance of insanity.' Galton was determined to leave his mark, but had found from his experiences at Cambridge that he could not compete in the same areas as others. He suffered from a deep-rooted sense of inferiority. Galton was an 'auto-didact' – a self-taught scientist, in the spirit of the times in which every respectable Victorian was an amateur scientist with a case of butterflies or a collection of skulls. But Galton was remarkable in that he chose obscure areas of study and took little or no interest in the work of others. He just began counting and measuring from scratch, evolving his own methods. He deliberately cast himself as an outsider. Throughout his life he tried to create his own, idiosyncratic areas of science in which to excel.

Galton's deep insecurity and need to assert his own genius underlay his initial decision to study heredity. Coming from a manufacturing background, he had now arrived in Victorian society, and sought implicitly to prove that his right to this position lay, not in whim or luck, but in hereditary traits which had inevitably propelled him to the top of his world. His eugenic theories made men like himself – the professional upper middle classes, the academics and scientists – the keystone of good breeding. They were the emergent new order.

Galton had religious doubts and even conducted one of his statistical tests on the efficacy of prayer. He surveyed the life spans of those who prayed regularly – including the Royal Family – to see if they lived longer, and horribly embarrassed his devout relations by publishing the results in which he concluded that, as regular prayer obviously did not lengthen life, it was useless.

Galton was never explicit about the reasons for his hostility towards conventional religion, but its emphasis on original sin seemed to trouble him particularly, which might be connected to guilt and shame within his own secretive, personal life. He was never forthcoming about himself; he hated introspection, preferring to look at life through a telescope or reduce its problems to sets of manageable statistics. But his marriage was unhappy – and, furthermore, sterile; Galton, the great advocate of good breeding, could have no children. He envisaged his compensation in terms of generations of perfect children created according to his eugenic theories. It is known that at some time on his early travels Galton put down his sextant and went in search of the pleasures of the flesh that statistics could not supply; he got a dose of venereal disease, to which he may have attributed his sterility. The clap – gonorrhoea – common among the proper middle classes of Victorian society who habitually frequented prostitutes, was traditionally associated with animal-like carnality; original sin. It would not be stretching the point to say that Galton's passion for eugenics stemmed from a deep sense of self-disgust. Eugenics elevated sex from indulgent pleasure to idealized, scientific act. Galton's wife was not keen on sex with him.

For him, eugenics was much more than a scientific theory; it assumed the nature of a secular religion. His last reservations were dispelled when he read his cousin Charles Darwin's *Descent of Man*. Instead of falling from a high estate, he told Darwin, man was 'rapidly rising from a low one'. Eugenics would greatly accelerate the process, breeding out the remaining barbarism of the human race: 'What Nature does blindly, slowly and ruthlessly, man may do providently, quickly and kindly.'

Before Galton's later publications, those who pondered good breeding fell into two camps. The social-Darwinists, on the one hand, believed that biology was destiny. There was no need to intervene scientifically in the breeding process, as the weak were doomed anyway. On the other hand, the strange emergent mixture of political and sexual radicals of the late nineteenth century were quick to embrace Galton's theories. They had been arguing that good breeding required the breaking down of social barriers to permit biologically sound sexual couplings.

Karl Pearson

In England, Galton's ideas were embraced by the Fabian socialist intellectuals and sexual radicals, those who, as in America, wished to use scientific arguments to attack the existing social and sexual barriers. Galton had no desire to eradicate any social boundaries, but it was among the thinkers of the left, including George Bernard Shaw, that his work found greatest favour. From these came his successor, Karl Pearson, who was to spread the gospel of eugenics in the twentieth century.

Although he styled himself a socialist radical, Karl Pearson was hardly liberal in his thoughts. Like many who came to preach the creed of eugenics, he came from a sexually repressed and spiritually dour background. A frigid and dogmatic character, he was christened Carl, but changed his name to Karl after developing a passion for German idealism and poetry, growing dewy-eyed over Goethe and enamoured of the thought of Fichte, an anti-Semite, who insisted that the good of the people was best expressed in the state to which their individuality should be subordinated. His socialist ideas did not include revolution; he saw the emergence of the perfect state as a consequence of education, a principle suited to his personal ambitions to be king of the dunghill rather than the one who destroyed it.

Pearson dreamed of marrying some strapping Rhine-maiden, but as he met few women of any description, let alone any German ones, he founded in 1885 the Men and Women's Club. Pearson had declared that the 'woman question' – female emancipation and women's rights – was the most important issue after socialism. The club would be a forum for frank discussions of male–female relations between representatives of the two sexes. Pearson, then a professor of mathematics at University College London, was approaching thirty and, like many Victorian men, had no experience or knowledge of women aside from the prostitutes he frequented. While the club did have an intellectual function, it also served as a useful dating agency for like minds, attracting some of the more outspoken and sexually adventurous women of the day. George Bernard Shaw noted, with glinting eye, the post-discussion opportunities that the club offered and applied for admittance. He was sniffily refused. It was at the club that Pearson met his wife.

Pearson elaborated and further defined Galton's theories of heredity arguing that after only a few generations of selective breeding the desired characteristics would be wholly dominant. Furthermore, he concluded that all physical and psychic characteristics in man were inheritable from bodily size to changes in mood. Galton and Pearson, who formed a father–son type relationship, seemed unlikely companions: the self-styled socialist and the comfortable upper-middle-class amateur. But if the impetus to Pearson's interest in eugenics had been to foster a society free of class barriers, this goal was now rarely revived in his rhetoric.

Pearson's fascination for eugenics became wholly nationalistic and increasingly conservative. He warned that 'Britain was ceasing as a nation to breed intelligence' (his evidence was that the car and the aeroplane had been invented by foreigners); this could only be redressed by breeding from the 'better stocks'. But the better stock, which was in description much like himself the professional, educated middle classes (though he also included the 'better sort of labourer' who had a 'clean body' and a 'sound if slow mind') had no economic incentives to beget children. Being responsible individuals, they assumed the financial burden for rearing, educating and maintaining their children. The irresponsible did the bulk of procreation. It was the case, he said in his influential public lectures, that 'the habitual criminal, the professional tramp, the tuberculous, the insane, the mentally defective, the alcoholic, the diseased from birth or from excess' were the parents of no less than half of each generation. Nor could education, which he had once advocated, stem the tide. One must breed intelligence. Charities for the children of 'Incapables' were 'a national curse and not a blessing'.

Like Galton's, his remedies were vague, but principally consisted of positive eugenic methods: financial incentives to encourage the desirable to have children. However, he did not rule out the necessity of negative eugenics; rather than encourage the desirable, it might be easier to suppress the undesirables. The state might have to intervene in the reproductive habits of 'antisocial propagators of unnecessary human beings'.

Pearson and his followers founded the journal *Biometrika,* through which they spread their gospel. He initiated the Biometric Laboratory whose only subjects for examination were statistics at University College. When Galton died in 1911, he left a large sum of money to the university in order to found a Galton Eugenics Professorship, which Pearson took. Pearson also became head of the new Department of Applied Statistics. In this expanded empire of eugenic theory the worker-bees processed large amounts of statistical data which Pearson then manipulated, interpreted and edited to reflect his beliefs. None of his students or colleagues were permitted to question or demur.

Eugenics, given a twist of nationalist panic, began to catch the public imagination in early twentieth-century Britain. Pearson's dire warnings on the state of the imperial bloodstock were taken most seriously by the press. Inspired by Galton and his successors, a national Eugenics Education Society was founded, with branches throughout the nation. Its function was to produce propaganda that would make the public more 'eugenically minded', to prepare them for the eugenics revolution. The society attracted the wealthy and influential. It was never short of money and was even able to produce films. Lecturers on the subject were sought after by every conceivable club and association, from health to the Women's Institute. A London woman who attended plays and concerts and conversed with writers, including H. G. Wells (who was developing alarming views on breeding) while pregnant, achieved celebrity by giving birth to 'England's first eugenic baby'. In London, the Bloomsbury drawing-rooms of the Ladies Emily Lutyens and Ottoline Morrell overflowed with eugenic thinkers. Each year brought a new spate of books on the subject and Galton was elevated to saintly status. With the advent of the First World War, interest died down, though the effects of the war were hotly disputed. Would the surviving men choose only the best and most beautiful women, thus making war a eugenic concept? Or would women be reduced to scrambling after anything male that was still in one piece?

Gregor Mendel and Negative Eugenics

Galton and Pearson had principally been advocates of positive eugenics – more people of the right sort. Now, in the early twentieth century, came the rise of negative eugenics – fewer people of the wrong sort. Negative eugenics was inspired less by the work of Pearson and company than by the long-ignored work of Gregor Mendel.

From an Austrian peasant family (not, according to the standards of Galton and his followers, a likely recipient of hereditary gifts), Mendel studied a battery of scientific subjects at Olmutz and Vienna universities before joining a monastery in 1843. He did this principally to have an environment in which to pursue his biological interests. For ten years he dedicated his life to growing peas in the monastery garden creating hybrid strains in order to find the laws that governed hereditary traits. It was slow work, and took some 30,000 pea-plants, all of which he analysed in terms of their tallness or shortness, or whether the peas they produced were wrinkled or smooth. Mendel concluded that the characters of the pea-plants were constituted by groups of 'elements'. The continuity of characteristics among the offspring of cross-bred plants was decided according to laws of probability; it depended how many elements of each characteristic their parents contained and communicated. Certain characteristics, emerging out of combining groups of elements, could disappear and reappear. They could not be easily dispersed, but were transmitted on.

When the monk published his conclusions in 1866, they were ignored. Science was engrossed by Darwin. The evolution of the species – change – was the rage; and change was also the theme of Galton and Pearson. Mendel's work showed not change, but stability; a genetic destiny that it was impossible systematically to breed out. When Mendel's work was rediscovered at the turn of the century, it caused much offence, particularly as it suggested that genetic evolution proceeded by a process of blending, and that the clear-cut good breeding so dear to Galton and Pearson was utterly wrong.

Now eugenicists began to turn their attention away from ways of breeding a better race from the good 'strain' towards isolating the undesirable hereditary traits which, they understood from Mendel's work, could not be bred out. Rather than studying the desirable types, they devoted their energies to identifying and labelling the undesirable. This was more fertile territory and found particular favour in America, where the race question, stirred by immigration and the emancipation of the negro slaves, began to trouble the white population.

Charles Davenport

Charles Davenport met and was inspired by Galton and Pearson. In 1904, he attracted huge funds to establish a station at Cold Harbour Spring outside New York for the experimental study of evolution. Here, Davenport initially did wholly respectable work on heredity in poultry and other animals according to the principles of Mendel; but he turned his attention to analysing human characteristics, and his prejudices emerged in all their glory.

Davenport once remarked that the most progressive revolution in history would be achieved if 'human matings could be placed on the same high plane as that of horse-breeding'. The good breeding stock of the nation was, typically, composed of people in his image. The multiple vices of the remainder could be seen to have specific roots in physiological and anatomical defects; so the 'pauperism' of the unemployed was due to the inefficiency of their physical and mental frames, and it was also possible to diagnose hereditary criminality and alcoholic tendencies by perfunctory examination. While he acknowledged that human breeding was complicated and a product of environment and blood, Davenport maintained that it was the racial 'protoplasm' of the individual that played the crucial role. Race was a question of nationality, which also determined behaviour. Of the current wave of immigrants, the Italians could be relied on for 'crimes of personal violence', the Hebrews were given to 'thieving', the Greeks were 'slovenly'. The great influx of alien protoplasm endangered previous American blood. The race would be 'darker in pigmentation, smaller in stature, more mercurial ... given to crimes of larceny, kidnapping, rape and sex-immorality'.

Davenport became the great American advocate of negative eugenics. He argued that as Mendel's work showed that characteristics would not easily break up, 'defective germ plasm' from foreigners would not be dispersed among the population but would remain, and be communicated through breeding with others, contaminating the good stock. Hence, he wanted a selective immigration policy, which would scan all individuals and their family histories for 'imbecile, epileptic, insane, crimi-

nalistic, alcoholic and sexually immoral tendencies.'
Meanwhile, he proposed that within the country they should
immediately start to prevent the procreation of the genetically
defective by state-enforced sterilization. By 1911, six states
had the measure on their statute books.

Davenport was yet another man with a puritanical background of sexual repression, religious zeal and family ambition. He was the archetypal WASP (White Anglo-Saxon
Protestant). Indeed, the burgeoning American eugenics drive
was led by WASPs. Davenport, like Pearson, was one of the
new generation of professional scientists who replaced the
amateurs exemplified by Galton. He had an overriding work
ethic, and in atonement for eschewing his father's example of
overwhelming religious piety threw himself into the worship of
science generally, and eugenics in particular. For him, also, it
was a secular religion for the new age. His mother, who
favoured science, was so keen to further his career that she regularly surveyed the death notices in the paper, keeping an eye
open for any scientific posts that might have suddenly fallen
vacant.

Davenport's ambitions were strictly middle-class; he was
obsessed with making enough money to live a respectable life
and was thrilled to be able to move into a sought-after neigh-
bourhood. He felt he had worked for what he had and deserved
it. The immigrants, on the other hand, and the defective, had
not and did not. Davenport bitterly resented the fact that his
taxes went to support them. He estimated that it cost the government, and by implication other respectable whites like himself, a hundred million dollars a year to support the insane, the
mentally deficient, epileptics, prisoners and paupers, not to
mention the swarms of immigrants, who were, he thought, of

such a bad standard that they must have been deliberately dumped by European powers plotting to weaken America. His eugenic theories were motivated by traditional WASP fears and resentments, principally of a financial and sexual nature.

Davenport had never enjoyed much sex himself and was rather fascinated by it. Sexual immorality was a characteristic of all forms of undesirables, particularly Jews, who he said 'showed the greatest proportion of crimes against chastity'. He concluded that 'innate eroticism', not financial need, was the cause of prostitution, of fits, and of criminality. Sexually-defective people were classed as 'feebly inhibited' because they could not master their desires. If they could not be segregated, they should be castrated.

Things had come a long way since Galton had peered through his sextant at the curvaceous form of a Hottentot girl, and Mendel had shuffled through his monastery garden at dawn, gently prising open the pods of his precious peas.

Davenport's indignation at the financial burden imposed by unsuitable types was shared by the public, their fears fostered by a stream of statistics from the American Eugenics Society and government agencies. The former pointed out that crime cost the average American family $500 per year, and that the 'majority of criminals have either defective intelligence, defective emotions or a combination of both defects'. Statistics, graphs and diagrams were the strategic weapons of the eugenics movement. Statistics had never been applied in this way before, to grade, package and define humans; it was the first time the public had been exposed to this sophisticated form of propaganda which thoroughly depersonalized and misrepresented their fellow humans. Then the IQ (Intelligence Quotient) test was also thrown into the fray.

Alfred Binet and intelligence tests

Intelligence tests were invented by a Frenchman, Alfred Binet. Binet evolved three vital rules to govern their use. First, the scores in an IQ test do not define anything innate; they do not tell you that somebody has a natural, inherited intelligence. Second, the scale is only of use in identifying children with learning difficulties, in order to help them; it is not to be used to measure normal children. Third, a low score does not indicate that a child is innately incapable.

In essence, all IQ tests measure is the participants' ability to perform an IQ test; to believe that they are a measure of something beyond that is presumptuous. Nevertheless, Binet's principles were adopted and shamelessly perverted by the eugenics movement. The tests that Binet had envisaged as identifying and assisting the educationally disadvantaged were seen as a means to weed out the 'feeble-minded' and 'witless'. In particular, two Americans, H. H. Goddard and Lewis M. Terman, introduced and developed their own versions of Binet's work.

Goddard was quick to propose that the feeble-minded identified by his tests should be prevented from breeding; he regarded all intelligence as inherited. 'We must learn,' he said, 'that there are great groups of men, labourers, who are but little above the child, who must be told what to do and shown how to do it ... there are only a few leaders, most must be followers.' He warned that the feeble-minded were 'multiplying at twice the rate of the general population.' He published photographs of a family – the Kallikaks – he claimed were a perfect example of the evil effects of thoughtless breeding. The faces of the supposedly stupid family looked twisted and depraved and had a considerable effect on public imagination.

Time has faded Goddard's photographs, now obvious as crude fakes.

It was Terman, a psychologist at Stanford University, who modified Binet's work to produce the model for nearly all subsequent IQ tests. He wanted everyone to be tested; the results of the tests would dictate which jobs the acceptable should be compelled to take. Terman, too, saw IQ tests as a means of identifying the inferior in order to eliminate them. In 1916, he wrote: 'In the near future intelligence tests will bring tens of thousands of these high-grade defectives under the surveillance and protection of society. This will ultimately result in curtailing the reproduction of feeble-mindedness and in the elimination of an enormous amount of crime, pauperism and industrial inefficiency.'

The IQ fashion reached a frenzied and fantastic zenith when, in 1921, the results of IQ tests carried out on two million American troops at the instigation of the American Psychological Association (APA) conclusively showed that the average American male was a moron with a mental age of around thirteen.

Rather than question the process, Robert Yerkes, the President of the APA and the nation's most prominent psychologist, used these ludicrous results to open a debate as to whether democracy was a viable system in a country where the voters were clearly so witless. Psychologists, inflamed with eugenic principles, were busy fantasizing about running society instead of questioning their motives.

The racial subtext of the tests helped to influence American immigration and social policy for many years. Yerkes demonstrated that, according to his data, fair-skinned, Nordic immigrants were more intelligent than dark-skinned Mediterranean types; Italians were more intelligent than Poles; and negroes, naturally, were at the bottom of the pile.

The tests were shambolic, the data were often perfunctory and the participants were rarely told what was happening and what the tests were about. What, if anything, the enormous pile of confused data has subsequently been shown to reveal is the significant effect environment has on 'intelligence', an effect which Yerkes would always choose to explain away in favour of his bigoted belief in racially-determined intelligence. There was a definite link between low scores and the participants being infested with hookworm. Hookworm is a sickness that thrives in impoverished communities, and the implication to a true scientific thinker would be that low scores were connected with poverty and thence with a lack of education. As far as Yerkes was concerned, the link demonstrated only that stupid people were likely to be poor, and poor, stupid people got sick; therefore, disease was a physical symptom of stupidity.

The tests also showed that racial integration produced similar scores among black and white; that blacks in Southern states, where discrimination was more acute, did worse; that the longer an immigrant had been in America, the better they performed in the test – yet all these factors, which clearly pointed to the effect of environment on so-called intelligence, were ignored.

Some prominent advocates of eugenics, like Alexis Carrell, Nobel Prize-winning surgeon and pioneering biologist, were openly pro-Nazi, and their work reflected not only a pragmatic interest in good breeding, but a quasi-mystical concern with race. Carrell, whose career rose and fell with the eugenics movement, was born in France in 1873. He emigrated to

America in 1904 and worked at the prestigious Rockefeller Institute until 1938. He finally died in France in 1944, disgraced as a Nazi collaborator. In 1939 he waxed lyrical on the subject of the mentally ill: 'Why do we keep all these useless and dangerous creatures alive? In Germany, the Government has taken energetic measures against the multiplication of inferior types, the insane and criminals. The ideal solution would be to eliminate all such individuals as soon as they proved dangerous.'

While supporting such negative eugenics, he possessed a mystical belief in the life force, in which he perceived a manifestation of the immortal qualities of race. In support of this belief, Carrell claimed to be able to breed what he asserted to be 'immortal cells'. Using extraordinarily complex surgical techniques which, for the outsider, smacked of ritual magic, he isolated cells from the hearts of chicken embryos and grew them in flasks. In an age before antibiotics, to grow cells for any duration, free of infection, was a considerable achievement. Of some sixteen 'cultures' commenced in January 1912, one survived until September, at which point Carrell announced that he had found the conditions under which the active life of a tissue of the organism could be prolonged indefinitely. Immersed in nutrients, and stringently protected from contaminating viruses – for which read racial impurities – the 'immortal' cells were propagated until 1922; a colleague, Eberling, claimed to have kept one culture alive until 1946. Carrell was hugely influential in the field of tissue culture, and the 'immortality' of the cells ensured his personal reputation and gave sanction to his views.

Other biologists were not able to repeat his success and over the years scepticism about his work grew. Finally, in the late 1950s, it was conclusively proved that indefinite culture of healthy cells was impossible, irrespective of how carefully they might be protected from viruses; only cancer cells are potentially immortal. It had been previously suggested by witnesses to Carrell's secret work, or those who had been permitted at some point to see the sacred 'immortal' cells, which were treated with distasteful reverence, that they were secretly replaced when they looked like wilting. Many of Carrell's assistants shared his ideological views; he was prepared to sacrifice his objectivity as a scientist to see his beliefs confirmed.

Eugenics and immigration

By the 1930s, despite sharing the views of their American colleagues, British eugenicists had been unable to have a comparable negative eugenics programme written into the laws of their own country. There was national anxiety about the weakening of stock caused by the proliferation of the mentally deficient, which Winston Churchill, then Home Secretary, described as a 'very terrible danger to the race', but the issue of immigration, which had been successfully manipulated by American eugenicists, was not a problem for Britain. Many eugenics campaigners in Britain were women, and none was more notable than Mrs Ellen Pinsent, who lobbied the government to prohibit breeding among the 'feeble-minded'. In 1912, under popular pressure, the government did introduce a mental deficiency bill which was passed with a large majority. It was intended to permit segregation of the mentally deficient, but after being ridiculed and attacked in the press for its authoritarian overtones, it emerged as a tolerant Act which did not impose mandatory segregation of undesirables. Sterilization and castration, to the disappointment of some, were not on the agenda.

The implicit belief in the hereditary nature of intelligence – the inherent good breeding of certain types, the triumph of nature over society's power to nurture – remained a part of conservative British thought. Long after the nightmares of the Nazi state demolished the eugenics movement, eugenic beliefs crept back in one disguise or another. Psychology, with its supposedly objective means of measuring human intelligence, was one such mask for individual prejudice, in the peculiar case of Sir Cyril Burt and his disappearing ladies.

Sir Cyril Burt, a firm believer in the hereditary nature of intelligence, worked as a research psychologist in the London educational system between 1913 and 1932. He was later instrumental, as a government adviser, in setting up the 11-plus educational structure, where children were tested, graded and assigned to one of three educational levels according to their perceived abilities. Using data he claimed to have collated in his twenty years as a research psychologist, Burt published an extensive series of IQ tests which appeared to supply incontrovertible evidence of the hereditary nature of intelligence. Burt was the first psychologist to be knighted, and became a pillar of the British establishment, holding the Chair of Psychology at University College, London. He died aged eighty-eight in 1971. So respected were his views that in 1969 an American scientist suggested that the current failure of special education schemes for racial minorities in America should be explained by the hypothesis that intelligence depended on racial heredity.

Important elements of Burt's assertions were based on research conducted on pairs of identical twins in the 1950s.

His data showed that the IQ of identical twins reared apart and in foster homes showed a remarkable similarity to the IQ of those reared together; environment had little effect on their innate intelligence.

Throughout the latter part of his career, Burt was occasionally pressed to supply more detailed information about his tests. He never bothered to provide any satisfactory answers, but his work was not generally doubted until after his death.

Leon Kamin

Then, in 1972, an American psychologist at Princeton University, Leon Kamin, noted considerable inconsistencies and gaps in Burt's methods and data. While generally referring those inquisitive about his methods to obscure theses by untraceable individuals who had once assisted him, Burt had specifically declared in one 1943 paper that a detailed description of his technique could be read in the degree essay of a Miss J. Maver, which was filed in the Psychological Laboratory, University College, London. No such document existed.

Kamin further pointed out that the results Burt had obtained from different tests on different sets of twins in the 1950s study were precisely the same, an impossible coincidence which until that point no one had remarked on. The realization that Burt had, at the very least, shamelessly adjusted his data to support his beliefs came as a considerable blow to his followers. It was impossible to check further by examining his personal records, as, acting on instructions from former colleagues, his house-keeper had burned them all after his death.

Supporters of Burt's work sadly acknowledged that it looked as if he had cooked the books to support his views. 'It is almost as if Burt regarded the actual data as merely an incidental backdrop for the illustration of the theoretical issues,' wrote one professor. They generously interpreted these inconsistencies as the errors of an old man; they did not believe, as Kamin now maintained, that Burt had cheated from the beginning and that all his published work was essentially fraudulent.

The plot thickened with the introduction of two mysterious ladies into the proceedings. These good ladies, Miss Margaret Howard and Miss J. Conway, were credited by Burt as being his collaborators in his published work. Efforts were made to trace the two ladies, whose names suggested a pair of reputable spinsters probably passing a genteel retirement in some seaside town. They could not be found, and in 1976, the *Sunday Times* reported that they did not exist, and probably never had existed. Burt had invented them.

Miss Howard and Miss Conway had, in their fictitious lives, been enthusiastic advocates of Burt's work. When Burt edited the *Journal of Statistical Psychology*, the dear ladies had been regular reviewers of his publications, for which they habitually had nothing but praise, and were prone regularly to eulogize the ideas of the great man. Their generosity did not extend to the work of his competitors and opponents, who were subject to vicious criticism.

When Burt ceased to edit the journal, the two ladies were patently overcome with grief, for they never wrote for it again. When the deception was revealed, it suddenly became obvious to those who had known him that every word written by Howard and Conway was unmistakably, shamelessly, Burt's. Why had they not seen it at the time? They believed a man of science was a man concerned with truth; but more, they agreed with Burt's ideas. They were prejudiced in favour of the heredity argument. They could not be objective.

Burt carefully preserved his friendship with these two useful alter egos. Their names became a familiar sound in the ears of the inquisitive and the doubting. When Burt was asked in 1969 how he had managed to conduct tests he claimed to have carried out on twins in the late 1950s, after he had retired, when he was without research facilities and was too old to have attempted such an extensive survey independently, he curtly replied that he had naturally delegated the work to the Misses Howard and Conway.

Surely Burt must have laughed as he invoked the two ladies yet again; his actions denote a degree of almost weary cynicism, the use of the names a well-worn private joke. He must have considered both critics and followers imbecilic. The fraud was not perpetrated merely because Cyril Burt wished to express his sense of humour, nor to prove the gullibility of the establishment, but because he considered that facts lacked the permanence of his beliefs. If the establishment was so insecure as to require the formal, token reassurance of evidence before it embraced theories that Burt held as fundamental principles, then he would oblige.

It was demonstrated in 1978 that Burt's figures for his studies on twins were taken from work he had published himself thirty years earlier. These figures had in turn originally been acquired, not by research, but by lifting and massaging data from a 1921 population survey. It was four years later that the British Psychological Society finally acknowledged that there was little foundation to Burt's work. While it can be impossible, armed with the most meticulous evidence, to convince people of a desperate truth they do not wish to acknowledge, one has only to articulate the most speculative but commonly held prejudice to achieve plausibility.

Eugenics and race

The German negative eugenics movement undoubtedly owed a debt to the early popularity of the American and British branches. The Americans were a particular encouragement, as they managed to have negative eugenics laws passed long before the Germans, who would have to wait until 1933, when Hitler was in power, for the first such law – the 'law for the restoration of the professional civil service,' which expelled all Jewish and half-Jewish individuals from the civil service – to be passed.

The intellectual roots of the Holocaust

The German movement was, from the beginning of the century, much more openly concerned with race, and specifically with anti-Semitism, than its counterparts, though the American soon caught up. There was a particular German word that encapsulated their precise concerns: *Rassenhygiene* (race hygiene). The first German eugenicists of this century were, like Galton, gentleman-scholars, amateurs. In 1905, one such amateur, Dr Ploetz, founded the Gesellschaft für Rassenhygiene (Society of Race Hygiene). Over the next twenty years, many academics and anthropologists involved themselves with the problems of 'miscegenation' and the ethics of killing those whose 'lives are not worth living'. A great many serious books on the subject were published. In 1923, Adolf Hitler could be found browsing through the pages of such volumes as *The Principles of Human Heredity and Race Hygiene*, a textbook by Professors

Lenz and Fischer. Fischer and others played integral parts in the international eugenics movement.

Fischer and the American Davenport were well acquainted. In 1929 Davenport, then President of the International Federation of Eugenic Organizations, sent Mussolini a memorandum written by Fischer on the subject of eugenics. 'Maximum speed is necessary,' it read; 'the danger is enormous.' In 1932, Dr Davenport invited Fischer to succeed him as President, but with the Nazis in the ascendant, Professor Eugene Fischer was becoming much too busy at home and declined the offer.

The precise horrors of the Holocaust have been well documented. Such industrialized killing requires the impetus of ideology to carry it on beyond the boundaries of human sensibility, after hate, blood-lust and even sadism have been exhausted. It was from the German scientific community that the Nazis derived such support. German scientists complied, *en masse*, with the Nazi eugenics programme. For German psychiatrists and anthropologists, biologists, anatomists, geneticists, ethnologists, eugenicists, human statisticians and behavioural scientists, the ascension of the Nazis to power brought state recognition of the value of their work. Ethnicity, race hygiene and good breeding were all part of the secular, though often foggily mystic, Nazi faith. With rare exceptions, the foremost German men of science co-operated at least to some degree with the authorities. Many were eager to offer their services, to underwrite ideologically the atrocities that were committed in the name of eugenics. Professor Fischer, Director of the Kaiser Wilhelm Institute of Anthropology, Human Heredity and Eugenics and Professor of Anthropology at the University of Berlin, who survived the war and lived to a contented old age, was reflecting general gratitude

Anti-Semitic Doctors

The rise of the Nazis caused some scientists to change their views in ways that they would later deny. Professor Lenz, Professor of Anthropology at the Kaiser Wilhelm Institute, once considered anti-Semitism to be groundless prejudice. In 1927 he published a book entitled *The Principles of Human Heredity and Race Hygiene*. In discussing the Jewish role in world revolution he considered the arguments of F. Kahn, whose book *The Jews as a Race and a People of Culture* was a standard text on the subject. 'Khan,' wrote Lenz, 'who values the Jewish revolutionary as a liberator of humanity, sees in these individuals "a specifically Jewish conception of the world and of historical activity." Many Jew-haters are of the opinion that the character of the Jews is subversive and negative. I do not think this is correct and believe that Jewish intellect, alongside the German, is the principal driving force of modern Western culture!' Nine years later, the passage in the new edition of the book had changed somewhat. It now read: 'Kahn ... sees in these individuals a "specifically Jewish conception of the world and of historical activity." The Jewish race has been depicted ... as a race of parasites. There is no doubt that the Jews constitute a grave handicap for their host nation ... a living creature develops better without parasites.' And so on, in the flavour of the times.

* * * * *

The American Eugenics Society

The Fitter Families Competitions were initiated in Kansas in 1920, sponsored by the American Eugenics Society. They soon sprang up nation-wide. They were held at fairs, in the 'human stock' section. Competing families had to submit their eugenic history and undergo blood tests and psychiatric examinations. At Kansas Free Fair in 1924, there were three prizes to be won, for small, medium and large families, and an additional medal for 'Grade A Individuals'.

for the marvellous opportunities science had recently enjoyed when he wrote in a newspaper in 1943: 'It is a rare and special good fortune for a theoretical science to flourish at a time when the prevailing ideology welcomes it, and its findings can immediately serve the policy of the state. The study of human heredity was already sufficiently mature to provide this when, years ago, National Socialism was recasting not only the state but also our ways of thinking and feeling ... the results of the study of human heredity became absolutely indispensable as a basis for the important laws and regulations created by the state.'

Professor Rudin, Doctor of Medicine, Honorary Professor and Director of Psychiatry at the Kaiser Wilhelm Institute, was, a few months earlier, similarly proud of the contribution academics had made to the Nazi murder machine, and took the opportunity to crow at those who had ever doubted that eugenics would find its theatre of operations: 'The results of our science had earlier attracted much attention (both support and opposition) in national and international circles. Nevertheless, it will always remain the undying, historic achievement of Adolf Hitler and his followers that they dared to take the first trailblazing and decisive steps towards such brilliant race-hygienic achievement in and for the German people ... the fight against parasitic alien races such as the Jews and gypsies and preventing the breeding of those with hereditary diseases and those of inferior stock.

Rudin was among the first to call for the compulsory sterilization of 'valueless individuals ... who were socially inferior psychopaths on account of moral confusion or severe ethical defects.'

Men like Rudin, considering themselves so fixed, so certain in the validity of their beliefs, provided the scientific justification for acts of mass torture, mass mutilation and mass murder. Indeed, in behaviour typical of the species, they even squabbled over who had ownership of which branch of undesirables. As a rule of thumb, the anthropologists busied themselves with rooting out and eliminating inferior non-Germans (Jews, Gypsies, Slavs and Negroes), while the psychiatrists rooted out and eliminated inferior Germans (schizophrenics, epileptics, imbeciles and psychopaths, including those with communist or anti-Nazi tendencies). There was enough work for everyone, but they still clashed from time to time. Should, for example, Gypsies who were also criminals be certified for sterilization or gassing on ethnic or psychiatric grounds? Of such delicate questions is the work of eugenics finally composed.

Nor were these men given specific instruction as to how they should think, or behave, by the authorities. They were not presented with detailed instructions for conducting mass extermination by Hitler or his associates. The multi-headed confusion of the Nazi state allowed such responsibility to be endlessly deferred to one department or another. They were simply encouraged to think as they saw fit. Wound up and then left to their own devices, these eminent men of science tottered gradually but inexorably down the path of genocide, while artfully managing to refrain from using precise words to describe the nightmare countryside they were passing through. They would not say what their destination was. It happened bit by bit, step by step. The result was that, in the case of the Final Solution, no one can, of course, remember whose idea it actually was. It arose out of multiple, duplicated acts, out of shared ideas and evasive conversations.

Consider this arch piece of euphemism, which should surely make advocates of politically correct language squirm. Some time in late 1938, possibly early 1939, a collection of German professors of psychiatry – de Crinis, Mauz, Polisch, Kihn and C. Schnieder – along with the esteemed anthropologist Professor Lenz, the mental hospital directors Drs Heinze, Falthauser and Pfannmüller, sat down and drafted a law permitting euthanasia. By the time they convened, the gassing-vans may well already have been rolling in and out of mental institutions, in which case the law was to apply retrospectively, or they may have been formulating the law in advance of the programme. The documentation, which includes the opinions of these eminent men, is undated. They were all agreed that such a law was urgently required, but one of their points of disagreement was over the title. Schnieder proposed a 'law for the granting of medical assistance to die'. It was not generous enough for Kihn, who countered with 'law for the granting of last aid'. Falthauser triumphantly came up with the most acceptable way to describe the process of systematic killing: 'law for the granting of special or specially assessed help'.

Silence, discretion, euphemism; the quiet meeting of like minds who understand without having to speak; 'one of the essential requirements for euthanasia,' ran a 1942 report, 'is that it should be as unobtrusive as possible.'

The actual executioners were doctors. From 1934, Professor Fischer was running training courses in eugenic sciences for SS doctors. They then learned the techniques of mass extermination as they went about the elimination of mental patients even before the war, gassing them with carbon monoxide in mobile units incorporated into vans or in special rooms at various mental hospitals. After some 94,000 had been disposed of, and another 100,000 starved to death, the programme was abandoned.

Euthanasia

The euthanasia of inferior German types was the only part of the sprawling race hygiene/eugenics programme to be halted due to public pressure. Loyal members of the Nazi public were puzzled to find out that their grandfathers, grandmothers, parents and other relatives had vanished, and many became suspicious after receiving a standard letter which ran: 'Dear [insert name]. We are sorry to tell you that your [insert relation], who had to be transferred to this Institution in accordance with measures taken by the National Defence Commissioner, died suddenly and unexpectedly here, of a brain tumour, on [insert date]. The life of the deceased had been a torment to [him/her] on account of [his/her] mental trouble. You should therefore feel that [his/her] death was a happy release. As this Institution is threatened by an epidemic at the present time, the police have ordered immediate cremation of the body. Any inquiries should be addressed to this Institution in writing, visits being for the present forbidden as part of the police precautions against infection ... '

The appearance of batches of identical obituary notices in local publications also alerted regional authorities who had not been informed of the euthanasia programme. The bodies of euthanasia victims were used for research. A Professor Hallervorden received at his own request 600 specimens of brain from the euthanasia stations. They were delivered in batches of 150-250 by a service calling itself 'The Limited Company for the Transport of Invalids in the Public Interest'.

'He [the physician] should go back to his origins, he should again become a priest, he should become priest and physician in one,' declared the Chief Physician of the Reich, Doctor Wagner.

And they did. They became priests of a cult of human sacrifice. Doctors, traditionally acquainted with the principle of inflicting minor destruction to cure major ills, were endowed with power over life and death, in order to cure the great eugenic disorder. They saw themselves as solving the great medical and psychiatric problems of their day. Despite the new, violent shock treatments, mental illness remained incurable, and psychiatrists had come to hate their patients. Professor Burger-Prinz, a psychiatrist in Heidelberg, wrote that as he strolled the wards one day, under the influence of mescaline, all the patients in his clinic turned into 'enormous worms'. Professors Binding and Hoche wrote in their book *The Sanctioning of the Destruction of Lives Unworthy to be Lived* that 'incurable idiots ... inspire terror in almost everyone'.

The killing of mental patients was only the beginning. Soon it was the turn of the Jews, the Gypsies and the Slavs. After Germany attacked Russia, the SS extermination squads found that they simply could not dispose of all the undesirables by shooting them. They sent for the death-doctors and their little gassing vans. 'My Dear little Wifey,' wrote the psychiatrist Mennecke, 'The day before yesterday a large contingent from our euthanasia programme moved to the eastern battle-zone. It consists of doctors, office personnel and male and female nurses.' The doctors were to supervise the extermination camps. Their vans went with them; they had been performing most satisfactorily, noted a civil servant from the Reich Head Security Agency. 'Since December 1941, using three vehicles, 97,000 persons have been processed without any defects occurring in these vehicles,' though as one had recently blown up they required a few 'technical modifications'.

The academics were consulted and pressed for their advice

and assistance at all stages of the genocide. Fischer, for one, attended conferences to discuss how best to deal with the millions of Jews and Slavs. Should they be dumped in Siberia? Or should they be 'scrapped through labour' – worked to death? Fischer warned against this last option if it included any possible improvement in living standards. These could 'easily lead to an increase in the birth rate'.

Quite apart from being given an opportunity to shape their world, scientists found that the concentration camps and prisons provided fertile conditions for testing eugenic theories. They also provided a consistent supply of skeletons and brains for collections. Doctor Mengele was interested in eyes. In the course of his genetic experiments at Auschwitz he used some one hundred pairs of twins, and the same number of families of dwarves and deformed people. If they did not die of the typhus or tuberculosis that was often experimentally inflicted on them, he killed them with injections to the heart and chopped them up for their organs. Eyes of different colours were extracted from the bodies of four pairs of murdered twins on one occasion; on another, a whole family of eight was killed for this purpose. The organs that Mengele did not want for his own research were packaged up and sent to grateful anthropological institutions nationwide, in packets marked 'War Material – Urgent'. After the war, many institutions would prove very quiet about the origins of their human specimen collections. Mengele set up his dissecting table in the crematoria, which gave him access to the concealed gold, jewels, gold teeth and wedding rings of the gassed victims. 'When will all this extermination cease?' asked his despairing slave assistant, Dr Nyiszli, one bloody day. His master looked up in some surprise. 'My friend!' said Dr Mengele, 'It will go on, and on, and on.'

Those scientists who did not travel all the way to the gas chambers and evaded Nuremberg, passing the De-nazification Tribunal (most, for lack of evidence which directly linked them to murders, were classified as 'fellow travellers'), and did not commit suicide (as at least seven prominent scientists did), returned to their academic work and declared that they knew nothing, saw nothing, heard nothing. They refused to discuss their former colleagues; they were bound together in their silence. In 1949, in passing judgement on one of their number whose wartime involvement with eugenics had cast a shadow on his professional career, a committee of German professors said that they could not 'consider a few isolated events of the past as marks of some unpardonable moral defect in a man who, in other respects, had honourably and courageously pursued his difficult path.'

Long after the war the ageing eugenicists could still be found in high academic positions in Berlin and Frankfurt, their views essentially unchanged. Some wrote their memoirs, which were notable for their lack of honesty. In Dr Fischer's published recollections, there was no mention of the Third Reich, or of the six million Jews.

In the deep freeze

Cryonicists used to be thought of as wackos: glittering-eyed technology freaks, playing in a morbid playground of pickled bodies, buckets of human antifreeze and vats of icy vapour, as megalomaniac underachievers plotting to revenge themselves on future generations by just being there, as super greedy consumers not content with gorging themselves in this life, or people who were simply so confused or frightened as to what death was that they would snatch at a chance to have a little longer to think about it.

Some cryonicists are still science fiction enthusiasts, but most are keen to stress how ordinary they are – bank managers, builders, computer programmers, professors and dictators. Since cryonicists have rejected death, they plan sensibly for the future, putting aside a little every week to ensure that their bodies will not be prematurely thawed because the maintenance money has run out. Cryonicists are often serious, reasonable converts, who say that they used to think the prospect of immortality was a sinister load of rubbish, but now they cannot understand how the 'deathists' can tolerate the thought of the grave. 'I thought it was a silly idea,' said a retired builder, 'then I went to Florida, saw all those ageing bodies on the beach, and said why should it end like this? Twenty years of wrinkling in the sun, then nothing. This is stranger than being frozen. Then the people who freeze you are really together and rational; they explain it just like an insurance policy. What's the point in not trying it? Either way you win. The worst that can happen is that it won't work, and you'll be dead. But that's what we're all geared up for anyway, and the hope that this isn't going to happen is going to make those last years a lot easier. And if it docs work – and there's every probability it will – I'll gain immortality. All it takes is a little faith now. After all, who would have thought that the same science that put men on the moon could produce the non-stick frying pan, if you see what I mean. I'm so confident that I've begun to worry how I'm going to make it through eternity financially.'

There are now companies that can help settle such anxieties;

the Reanimation Foundation in Lichtenstein, for example, will invest your money against the day of your return.

Techniques

At the moment of clinical death, the cryonicist becomes a cryonaut, the flesh super-cooled in liquid nitrogen, in anticipation of a time when doctors will make available to the public the techniques to restore the dead to life and, once they are alive, will give health to the sick, youth to the aged, and will elevate all peoples to a supreme intellectual state and maintain them as immortals.

All this remains at present, theoretical. It would be murder for others to freeze you while you are still alive and, since the process is speculative, you are advised to make the most of this life, just in case.

The process is quite simple; it is technologically enhanced embalming. Once certified clinically dead, you should be taken to the coldest available room and, if possible, circulation should be maintained using a heart/lung machine, by artificial respiration or by massaging the heart, until your body temperature has been gradually lowered by the use of ice packs.

If you are a member of a cryonics society, your relatives should by now have called them, and with luck their corporate employees (but most probably volunteers) will be on their way in a specially converted ambulance, in which your corpse can be preserved until it has reached the society's operating table. If you have opted for the expensive course of full body freezing your blood will be drained and the cadaver perfused with a solution of glycerol and other preservatives such as sodium chloride, dextrose, disodium glycerophosphate, heparin, noradrenalin, penicillin and sodium bicarbonate. If you have chosen only to have your head preserved, they will cut it off. Surgeons may perform the operations, but speed is essential so enthusiastic amateurs have been trained to stand in for orthodox surgical staff. Wrapped in plastic and packed in carbon dioxide your body will then be taken to a long-term storage facility – probably in the United States – where it will be lowered into a steel flask of liquid nitrogen. At minus 196 degrees, your body will await the moment when technology will have caught up with your ambitions and you can be revived.

Perhaps you may have to wait 200 years, but there is little doubt that at some point scientists will be capable of reviving a corpse, after a fashion. But before introducing the animating spark they will have to repair or replace much of your tissue. In addition to any damage suffered at death – cancer, gunshot wounds, the impact of a car, old age – the body decays from the moment circulation ceases. Critical brain damage is sustained. Supercooling also tears the cells as ice crystals form inside the tissue, and there is no known way in which the poisonous cocktail of preservatives might be expelled from the body.

Robert Ettinger

Such obstacles to eternal life, allied to enormous cost and a lack of positive publicity have assured the cryonics movement of a mixed reception. Since its prime mover and high priest, Robert Ettinger, published his bestselling cryonic scripture, *The Prospect of Immortality*, in 1964, the movement has had its ups and downs, its own freezings and thawings. But there is currently a resurgence; several hundred people have signed up for the programme, and the bodies or heads of some 50 cryonauts have already begun their cold voyage into the future.

'It is like a horror film, in a way,' recalls one man who has seen inside a cryonics vat. 'I looked inside the tank when it was being topped up with liquid nitrogen. As the swirls of vapour cleared away, you could see the patients hanging down below on wires in polythene bags.'

In the 1960s, Ettinger, an unassuming Michigan professor, argued that advances in cryobiology – the freezing of living cells, of blood serum, sperm and tissue – were so encouraging that it was then theoretically possible to freeze people at their clinical deaths. Surveying the rapid advances in technology that had within a few years led to computers and the first primitive robots, he predicted that when resuscitation techniques were widely available cryonics would usher in a technically sophisticated and culturally pragmatic Golden Age in which mankind would be raised to the level of the Olympians.

Such a dramatic vision, wrote Ettinger, should not only be the aspiration of every rational self-interested human, but also the goal of a humane and altruistic society. He reasoned that fear of extinction governs the behaviours of both aggressors and victims; if elimination of oneself or one's enemies were almost impossible, might not a freezer-culture remove even the possibility of nuclear war? And on a more petty level, might not individual acts of malice or greed be rejected in the knowledge that, sentenced to eternal life, one would never escape the consequences of one's actions.

'The prospect of immortality,' wrote Ettinger, 'should provide a strong damper on rash and impetuous action and antisocial behaviour. National leaders will want to preserve their own skins and will be forced to take a longer view. A temporary advantage will become unimportant. When immortality has actually been realized there will be very salutary effects on interpersonal behaviour ... there may well be a Golden Age of morality and ethics.'

It would be possible, he hoped, 'to make the punishment fit the crime. Culprits may be made to suffer all that their victims have suffered, and to make complete restitution.'

This visionary world will make childbirth redundant. 'At present, of course, many women will not admit the ordeal is disgusting, and many even insist it is "beautiful". But this is obviously just a psychological trick, making a virtue of necessity. One might just as well claim our methods of waste elimination are beautiful.'

Nor was there any reason to worry about overpopulation, or consumption. The machines that rebuild us will create from the atoms of the air anything that we desire.

It was not necessary to wait for the means for resurrection to become available, only to know that it was possible to freeze; and Ettinger called for immediate instigation of a mass freezer programme, speculating that a demand for immortality would then force the market to produce the requisite technology. At first he envisaged that only rich and enlightened individuals would be frozen; but he assumed that soon all governments must follow the same course, and that soon so many people would have opted to be frozen at death that 'the frozen will constitute an enormous body of influence which must be duly recognised and represented.' The interests of the dead would spawn legislation and the future rights of those who had lived would shape the choices of their offspring. 'The people in freezers should also be protected by family loyalties, and by a tradition that recognizes that each in his turn must become frozen and helpless, dependent upon the goodwill and law-abiding character of his successors.' In this way, with great resources committed, society would be compelled to acknowledge as authentic the ambitions of the cryonauts. All that was needed was for people of courage to commence the programme.

Ettinger was comforted by research into parallel fields, some of it highly speculative. Certainly living cells could be frozen and thawed; Ettinger was particularly drawn to the work of Jean Rostand, a French biologist who had used glycerol to freeze frog sperm. In the late 1940s fowl sperm had been frozen, and in the 1950s the United States Navy Tissue Bank had begun freeze-drying human tissue. The British physiologist Sir Alan Parkes also used glycerol to preserve living cells, and later froze, and revived (briefly for the most part) rats, mice and dogs. He thought that his work would have applications for artificial insemination and organ transplantation. Fervent cryonicists would repeat these experiments, in their own freezers and fridges. Years later, the relative of a frozen cryonaut paid a visit to the glum storage facility, where her loved one was suspended in a steel tube in the corner. 'There was an ice-cream container on top of one of the capsules,' she recalled, ' the President said he had a six-week-old fetus in it. He was experimenting with freezing to see if it could be brought back to life.'

Supercooling
None of the progressive cryobiological experimenters had considered supercooling; the mammals had been frozen in ice, carbon dioxide or just held in freezing water; and they had, of course, all been alive when they were chilled.

But by the early 1960s it was apparent that extraordinary,

even miraculous, things happened at supercooled temperatures, and that this authentic science of cryogenics would have lucrative commercial applications. It was known for example, that submerged in liquid nitrogen or helium at cryogenic temperatures, between −196 and −320 degrees, some metals would produce strong magnetic fields without consuming electricity; civilisation had always associated life with heat, but now, at a point below zero where all was cold and dead, a spark of energy was spontaneously generated. The cryonicist, looking for scientific reason for his hope in freezing, could comfort himself with mysticism.

Ettinger's book was reprinted several times. The inspiration of the movement, he was not the dynamic public leader it required, though he did found the Cryonics Society of Michigan, and promoted research into 'life extension, gerontology, ageing research, cryonics, futurism, death and dying.' Those responsible for founding the dozen cryonics branches that sprang up in the latter part of the 1960s were a mixture of the middle class, science fiction enthusiasts and financial opportunists who thought that cryonics was the industry of the future.

Cryonics societies charged a fee for membership, though many members of the public simply subscribed to the prolific publications: *Long Life*, *The Life Extension Journal*, *Happy Ever After*, *The Cryonaut*. These contained encouraging reports on how Soviet scientists were reported to have frozen embryos, transplanted the organs of dogs into monkeys and isolated rejuvenating hormones that wiped the wrinkles away. They would also contain handy tips on DIY prefreezing surgery ('Which artery counts?' 'A basic perfusion toolbox; look no further than your local hardware store!' 'How to mix antifreeze ... ') and offer advice on the legalities of being frozen: 'Make sure it's all on paper; oblige the survivors to carry out your wishes AND PAY THE STORAGE BILLS. Remember; defaulters don't make it to the Future.'

Meetings provided the opportunity for members to discuss progress in the field, and to suggest ways that the message could be spread. The founders of societies did anticipate that they would become very rich, but for the present were content to present the societies as financially disinterested organisations, until the first man was frozen; then they hoped for a stampede.

'Do you have a good life full of the best our civilization can offer?' read their publicity. 'You've worked hard all your life to earn those rewards; the simple pleasures of vacations, of home comforts, of being with the beautiful woman you love. Do you ever want this to end? We think that your answer will be no. Then why have you not yet signed up for eternal life? By subscribing to our society you will have a unique opportunity to contribute towards the single greatest advance in science; the indefinite extension of your life. And one day, in a state of inexhaustible youthful vigour, you will live the life that you, and you alone, chose, a life in which you will be unfettered by physical limitations and unburdened by the prospect of the grave. Talk to us about the technological miracles that will keep you forever young.'

It was hoped that those opting for freezing would pay a capital sum for the operation, perfusion and their steel 'Forever Flask'; there would be rental and maintenance charges for the relatives to bear. Members of societies were encouraged to take out large insurance policies to cover the initial cost.

Though hundreds of Americans joined cryonics societies,

nothing further happened. People sat and talked about freezing each other, and how they would spend the future centuries; they evolved a language without suggestions of death or finality, calling the frozen the 'suspended'.

One problem was that cryonics appealed to a young generation. The majority of followers were white, male and affluent. They were often keen 'survivalists' with an interest in guns and nuclear fallout shelters under their houses. They were not likely to die for years. When cryonicists did die, their relatives often prevented their bodies from being frozen. Interest waned. Then, in 1967, one society froze the first man.

There is some dispute over who the first 'corpsicle' (as conventional doctors dubbed the cryonauts) actually was. Some claim that first suspension took place on 12 January 1967, on Harold Greene, a retired psychiatrist. More claims are made for James Bedford a retired psychology professor, who was also said to have been frozen that month. The latter claim was endorsed by Robert Nelson, an electronics engineer turned prominent cryonicist, who in 1967 published his book *We Froze the First Man*.

The publicity generated a quick spate of freezings. Some found the transformation from theory to practice hard to stomach, and the societies did not always acquit themselves well, their promised gleaming facilities proving little more than kitchen cupboards and damp crypts.

Sunrise Cryonics

Sunrise Cryonics, for example, was thought one of the better equipped societies. By 1966, it had drummed up about 100 members; these were soon tired of waiting. But after Greene, or Bedford, was frozen the society quickly received applications to freeze two bodies; a third was allowed to thaw when the relatives changed their minds. The society did freeze five bodies; but the founders were so desperate for funds that they stretched their members' patience when they agreed to freeze a man who had been buried and had to be exhumed. And the fabric of the society decayed further over the question of where the bodies should be stored. The serious cryonicists were determined that they should be seen as normal people, whose beliefs did not conflict with Christian ideas. It was a matter of respectability for some that orthodox funeral services were conducted, though they could not always take the steel flasks through the church doors; and most preferred that their relatives be stored in suitably inert company. The society therefore leased a crypt in a cemetery; but the cemetery's owners soon bowed to complaints from local residents and demanded that the capsules be removed. Some relatives claimed that this was the fault of the society's officers who kept bizarre hours, entering the cemetery at night to top up the nitrogen levels. In general, the society's members perceived themselves as quite reasonable, while those who ran the organisation were freaks, an impression strengthened when the founders proposed removing the bodies to an industrial warehouse. 'I saw the founder,' recalled one member, 'in this office, really empty, not even a chair for me to sit on. He was reading a science fiction story, and he had this pile of comics on his desk. He hadn't shaved for a week. I complained about my wife being put in an old furniture store and he looked at me and said, "We're not sending them to an old furniture store we're sending them to another planet." Then he gave me a new price for the maintenance. Much higher than agreed. I must have looked green because he said, "Pay or decay!" and went back to his comic.'

That society collapsed into a number of redundant splinter

groups; and in the end it was left to individual relatives to look after the storage of their own loved ones. Some put them in their cellars or garages.

In the 1970s there were only a few freezings, and these were often tragic gestures by hopelessly distressed relatives; a young mother who died of leukaemia; the brain of an infant battered to death.

The movement struggled to overcome bad publicity. In 1970, Terry Harris, a Los Angeles businessman paid the Cryonics Society of California $10,000 to freeze his mother, who had died of cancer. Harris later paid for his father to be frozen alongside her. Two years later, the society froze its first child, a seven-year-old girl who had died of cancer; it was then thought to have up to a dozen 'corpsicles' in a vault.

But ten years later the society went bust and anxious relatives tried to find out where and in what condition the corpses were. An investigative reporter located nine of them in a suburban crypt in Los Angeles; some bodies were decomposing in wooden packing crates; others were inside steel flasks, but the liquid nitrogen had evaporated. The president of the society was by then working as a television repairman.

Embryonic cultures often benefit from the conversion of sober celebrities. But the figures interested in cryonics confirmed the public suspicion of a movement for eccentrics. Walt Disney was constantly rumoured to be in suspension beneath the Californian desert (though his family apparently insisted he be cremated); Howard Hughes was also said to have had a fascination for cryonics, and Salvador Dali was another thought to have opted for freezing. Relatives of the Nicaraguan dictator Anastasio Somoza took his remains to a Florida cryonics organisation, which reluctantly turned them down because there was not much left of Somoza, and they feared that keeping the residue on ice would provoke a terrorist attack. During the recent Gulf Crisis, rumours began to circulate that representatives of the Iraqi dictator Saddam Hussein had approached an American cryonics society to discuss freezing Hussein's sperm or cell tissue from which a clone might be made.

And then there was the high expense; in 1976 the estimated cost of preparation and indefinite storage for one person was $50,000. It would take a generation for those believing in cryonics to reach the level of financial comfort at which they would feel able to take out the necessary policies. By the early 1980s cryonics looked defunct. But recent work on genes and cloning has given the cryonicists hope. This has gone some way to reducing costs.

Decapitation after death ('neurosuspension') is half the cost of full body freezing. Cryonicists now think that by the time clinical resurrection is possible we may in any case have no need of limbs, but will be super-intelligent jellies, governing our surroundings through a web of wires hooked into the brain. Many of the recent converts to cryonics are young computer enthusiasts who imagine that their personalities will be downloaded onto a mainframe system. The Alcor Life Extension Institute has frozen 10 bodies and 17 heads.

Most of the new cryonics organisations were established on the basis that the putative cryonaut would pay for their own suspension in advance. In 1994, Alcor was said to have 350 people throughout the world who had signed up at $324 a year (half-price for a second family member) to be frozen on death, among them Timothy Leary, the 1960s Harvard 'Messiah of LSD'. Alcor had also suspended a number of pets, principally dogs, at lower rates.

There are said to be more than 20 Britons signed up to the Alcor programme. A halfway house has been opened in Sussex to chill the bodies before transportation to the United States. The British society members must be prepared to perform suspensions if an American medical team cannot be imported in time. 'It's basically heart surgery with a bit of brain thrown in,' commented one member. By 1993, they had only actually frozen one man; then the family had second thoughts, and he was thawed.

The movement continues to generate controversy. Alcor recently moved its operations from California to Arizona, partly to escape Californian bureaucracy, which led to the arrest of five employees after an eighty-seven-year-old woman was decapitated ready for freezing. The coroner of Riverside County accused Alcor of removing the head of Mrs Dora Kent before she was dead; he wished to examine the head, but the company refused to hand it over, since it would have had to be defrosted.

Another reason for moving base was the fear of Californian earthquakes. Alcor's patients cannot leave their beds. One of them is James Bedford, perhaps the first cryonaut, who was handed over to Alcor three years ago.

Cryonicists know that they will not be taken seriously until one of their members is successfully revived. But this will probably take much longer than Ettinger ever envisaged; mortality provides the basis for most ethical and economic structures in society, and the elimination of death is not an immediate priority. The clear-headed accept that upon resuscitation they are unlikely to retain the personalities they are now so attached to, and would rather concentrate on extending this life. The longer we live, the more illnesses we encounter.

Each advance in gerontology creates a myriad of problems it takes decades to conquer.

'They're not doing the right kind of pure research just now', acknowledges one cryonicist, 'Everything has got to have some spin-off, some kind of so-called benefit to mankind. Until people start thinking about themselves seriously, we aren't going to get the first man revived. They've got to see it as the great voyage, and save my frozen ass. I got invested $100,000 says I live; my wife is angry about those missed holidays, the old car. I got to win the argument (not that I want her to join me in the flask).'

Index